DATE DUE

DEC 0 8 1993			
JAN 0 1 1995			
MAY 2 2 2002			
			PRINTED IN U.S.A.
GAYLORD			

The Macrophage

The Macrophage

NANCY N. PEARSALL, Ph.D.

Acting Instructor
Department of Microbiology
University of Washington School of
  Medicine
Seattle, Washington

RUSSELL S. WEISER, Ph.D.

Professor of Immunology
Department of Microbiology
University of Washington School of
  Medicine
Seattle, Washington

Lea & Febiger

PHILADELPHIA, 1970

ISBN 0-8121-0278-9

Library of Congress Catalog Card Number: 77-85844

PRINTED IN THE UNITED STATES OF AMERICA

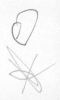

Preface

THE UBIQUITOUS phagocytic cells that we know as macrophages vary in many of their characteristics, depending on their location, physiological state, and function. Although Metchnikoff appreciated many of their potentialities nearly a century ago, most early investigators regarded macrophages primarily as scavenger cells. Research in many fields has made it increasingly obvious that macrophages do, in fact, have a multitude of important functions above and beyond their ability to scavenge and dispose of effete cells and extraneous matter.

Several decades ago it was realized that macrophages are the chief agents of antimicrobial cellular immunity. Only during the past few years has the importance of the macrophage-cytophilic antibody system in cellular immunity been appreciated. The maturation of monocytes to macrophages, then to epithelioid cells, and finally to giant cells, has been described both *in vivo* and *in vitro*. The contribution of this sequence of events to cellular immunity is not fully apparent but is of great interest.

Recent research has led to an awareness of the extensive synthetic capabilities of macrophages. It has been shown that these cells can synthesize interferon, components of complement, and numerous other biologically active substances, including a wide array of enzymes.

Macrophages are important in allograft rejection. They function in delayed sensitivity reactions and in the pathogenesis of autoimmune diseases. They are probably often essential to antibody formation by their activities of trapping and processing antigen, and perhaps by virtue of the activity of their ribonucleic acid. In addition, macrophages are able to detoxify both exotoxins and endotoxins, as well as other injurious compounds.

Thus, macrophages have emerged from their historical role as simple scavenger cells to take their place, with lymphocytes, as mobile cells with a wide spectrum of functions of primary importance to body economy.

The possible relationships between macrophages and lymphocytes, and between macrophages and other cell types, remain controversial. However, it is probable that one vital function of macrophages is to regulate the proliferation and differentiation of other cell types, and, conversely, that other cells contribute to macrophage homeostasis.

Recent rapid advances in research concerning macrophages have resulted in a tremendous increase in the literature, scattered throughout a wide variety of publications. The object of preparing this monograph is twofold: first, to consolidate available information in order to provide a comprehensive characterization of the macrophage for those unfamiliar with it; and, second, to review some of the most recent work in this area for the benefit of those who are already familiar with the field. Wherever possible, reviews are quoted. Many recent findings, not summarized elsewhere, are reviewed in detail. It is hoped that the references cited will provide a point of departure for gaining further information on subjects of special interest to the reader.

Even though much is known about the macrophage and its functions, many problems of great interest remain unsolved. For example, consideration of the control mechanisms which operate in the proliferation and differentiation of macrophages offers a challenge for future research. In addition, the molecular events concerned in macrophage-cytophilic antibody activity are of the utmost importance and are incompletely understood. These and similar problems provide promising areas for further investigation.

There are many who have participated, directly or indirectly, in the preparation of this monograph. Although it it not possible to thank each one individually, our debt to them is great, and we are appreciative of their contributions. We are grateful to our colleagues who have read portions of the manuscript and offered valuable suggestions. Special thanks are due to Dr. Q. N. Myrvik and Mrs. E. S. Leake, not only for their criticisms of the manuscript, but also for a number of electron micrographs.

Seattle, Washington   NANCY NEVILLE PEARSALL
                                                         RUSSELL S. WEISER

Contents

Chapter 1.   Introduction   1

   Summary   3

Chapter 2.   The Structure of Macrophages   5

   A. Monocytes   5
   B. Peritoneal Macrophages   6
   C. Alveolar Macrophages   9
   D. Splenic Macrophages   11
   E. Macrophages of Lymph Nodes and Thymus   11
   F. Liver Macrophages (Kupffer Cells)   12
   G. Central Nervous System Macrophages (Microglia Cells) ..   13
   H. Macrophages of Other Organs and Tissues   13
   I. Epithelioid Cells and Giant Cells   14
   Summary   16

Chapter 3.   The Phylogeny and Ontogeny of Macrophages   17

   A. Phylogeny   17
   B. Ontogeny   18
   Summary   19

Chapter 4.   Sources, Maturation, and Life Span of Macrophages   21

   A. Bone Marrow Stem Cells as Progenitors of Macrophages ..   21
   B. Blood Monocytes as Circulating Immature Macrophages ...   22
   C. Other Possible Sources of Macrophages   23
   D. The Controversy Concerning Lymphocyte-to-Macrophage Transformation   27
   Summary   30

Chapter 5.   Macrophages and Cellular Homeostasis   31

   A. General Theories Concerning Homeostasis   31
   B. Factors Influencing Macrophage Proliferation and Differentiation   34

1. Lipids 34
2. Endotoxins 34
3. Monocytogenic Hormone 35
4. Other Agents 36
C. Cellular Interrelationships 36
1. Macrophage and Plasma Cell 36
2. Lymphocyte and Macrophage 37
3. Macrophage and Fibroblast 37
4. Polymorphonuclear Neutrophil and Macrophage 39
5. Macrophage and Macrophage 40
Summary 40

Chapter 6. Macrophage Metabolism 41

A. Metabolic Requirements in Vitro 41
B. Energy Sources 42
1. Peritoneal Macrophages 42
2. Alveolar Macrophages 43
C. Synthesis of Enzymes 43
1. Peritoneal Macrophages 44
2. Alveolar Macrophages 45
3. Blood Monocytes and Tissue Macrophages 46
D. Synthesis of Lipids 50
E. Synthesis of Interferon 52
F. Synthesis of Serum Proteins 53
G. Relation of Metabolic Activities to Cellular Functions 53
Summary 55

Chapter 7. Phagocytosis by Macrophages 57

A. Uptake of Extracellular Materials by Macrophages 57
B. Mechanisms of Phagocytosis 58
C. Phagocytic Energy Requirements 61
D. The Role of Humoral Factors in Phagocytosis 62
E. Reticuloendothelial Function 64
F. Additional Factors Known to Influence Phagocytosis and
      Reticuloendothelial Function 65
Summary 69

Chapter 8. Functions of Macrophages 71

A. Scavenger Activities 71
1. Cytophilic Opsonins as an Aid in Scavenger Activities .. 71
2. Disposal of Tissue Debris and Effete Cells 72
3. Action of Macrophages on Sensitized Erythrocytes 74
4. Wound Healing 76

B. Regional Activities 77
  1. Peritoneum 77
  2. Lung 77
  3. Central Nervous System 79
  4. Lymphoid Tissue 79
  5. Testes 80
  6. Skin 80
  7. Bone 80
C. Additional Functions of Macrophages 80
  1. Detoxification 80
  2. Inactivation of Thromboplastin 81
Summary 82

Chapter 9. The Role of Macrophages in the Antibody Response 83

A. Contributions of Macrophages to the Antibody Response
     in Vivo 83
  1. Antigen Trapping 84
  2. Antigen Processing 85
  3. Antigen Storage 88
  4. Influence on Cellular Homeostasis 89
B. Contributions of Macrophages to Antibody Production
     in Vitro 89
  1. Studies with Whole Cells 89
  2. Studies with Subcellular Components 90
Summary 91

Chapter 10. Antibodies Cytophilic for Macrophages 93

A. Characteristics of Antibodies Cytophilic for Macrophages .. 94
B. Nature of Macrophage Receptors and the Cytophilic-Binding
     Reaction 97
C. Significance of Antibodies Cytophilic for Macrophages 99
Summary 100

Chapter 11. The Macrophage in Delayed Sensivity 101

A. Studies in Vivo 103
B. Studies in Vitro 108
Summary 113

Chapter 12. Macrophages and Acquired Cellular Immunity 115

A. Anti-tissue Cellular Immunity 116
  1. Allograft Immunity 116
     a. Studies in Vivo 117
     b. Studies in Vitro 119

2. Immunity to Autochthonous Tumors 121
3. Autoimmune Diseases 123
4. Theoretical Aspects of Anti-tissue Cellular Immunity ... 123
B. Antimicrobial Cellular Immunity 124
1. Mycobacterial Systems 127
a. Tuberculosis 127
b. Leprosy 130
2. The Listeria System 135
3. The Salmonella System 136
4. Other Antimicrobial Systems 137
5. Ultrastructural Responses of Macrophages to Intracellular
Microbes 139
6. The Relation of Delayed Sensitivity to Antimicrobial
Cellular Immunity 143
7. Theoretical Aspects of Antimicrobial Cellular Immunity 143
Summary 145

Chapter 13. Macrophages in Disease 147

A. Infectious Diseases 147
B. Metabolic Diseases 148
C. Intercellular Imbalances 149
D. Macrophages and Neoplasms 150
E. Possible Contributions of Macrophages to the Pathogenesis
of Disease States 150
Summary 151

Bibliography 153

Index 197

Chapter 1
Introduction

THE TERM *macrophage* will be used in the following pages to define a ubiquitous large mononuclear cell type characterized by the ability to phagocytize particulate material and to store vital dyes. Among the many names that have been used to designate cells fulfilling these criteria are the following, for which complete references may be found in the review by Sacks (1926): clasmatocytes (Ranvier, 1900), adventitial cells (Marchand, 1901), Kupffer cells (Ribbert, 1904), rhagiocrine cells (Renaut, 1907), mononuclear leukocytes (Aschoff, 1924), pyrrol cells (Goldmann, 1909), histiocytes (Kiyono, 1914; Maximow, 1924), and reticular cells (Aschoff, 1924). In addition, Hortega cells of the central nervous system are generally regarded to be macrophages (de Asúa Jiménez, 1927), and septal cells of the lung are sometimes classified as macrophages (Robertson, 1941). This list, although incomplete, illustrates the great diversity of cells defined as macrophages. The diversity of this cell type accounts for many of the controversies which have arisen during investigations conducted over the past hundred years.

Near the turn of the century, Metchnikoff (1905) discussed the concepts of immunology current at that time, including his own avant-garde ideas concerning phagocytosis. He reviewed some of the earliest reports on phagocytosis by mammalian leukocytes, published by Grawitz in 1877 and 1881, and also discussed his own experiments on macrophages, which began during the same decade.

Metchnikoff was a zoologist who was primarily interested in determining the function of the mesoderm. Although at the time it was widely accepted that the ectoderm supplies the cutaneous layers and the entoderm the digestive organs of multicellular animals, the function of the mesoderm was completely obscure. The work of Metchnikoff with sponges and other lower animals revealed that ameboid cells of their mesoderm could actively ingest, and subsequently digest, foreign materials. Even though Metchnikoff was not medically trained, he had encountered Cohnheim's writings on pathology and had been particularly impressed with the descriptions of "ameboid cell" infiltrations and with his theories on inflammation in the human. He was struck by the similarities between leukocytes in inflammatory exudates of higher animals and phagocytic ameboid cells of the echinoderms, and hypothesized that cells of this type have the important function in body defense of ingesting and digesting extraneous material. To test this hypothesis, he inserted rose thorns into the transparent bodies of starfish larvae. Metchnikoff postulated that if ameboid phagocytes are important in defense they should accumulate at sites of injury. Much to his delight, as he watched the transparent animals, masses of ameboid cells collected around each inserted thorn. Since the starfish larvae had neither blood vessels nor a nervous system, he concluded that this cellular exudation must represent a primitive basic defense mechanism. Metchnikoff speculated that the ingestion and digestion of extraneous materials by human ameboid phagocytes represents an analogous mechanism which has been retained throughout evolution because it offers a highly efficient defense against invasion by foreign agents.

Virchow (1885) was interested in, and favorable to, Metchnikoff's proposal that phagocytes in an inflammatory exudate function as agents to destroy invading microorganisms, even though during his time pathologists generally accepted the view that cells which ingest bacteria play a harmful role in infection because they serve as vehicles of microbial dissemination. This concept had developed because microbes could be seen within motile phagocytes, but no evidence had been found that they were destroyed intracellularly.

Metchnikoff (1884a) was able to show that materials are digested within phagocytes of various species and that engulfment of anthrax bacilli (1884b) by phagocytes of vertebrate animals leads to, in his words, "a desperate struggle" between bacilli and the ameboid cells.

The principal tenet of "the theory of phagocytes," formulated by Metchnikoff, was that phagocytes are solely responsible for immunity to harmful agents. This led to a controversy between supporters of this theory and proponents of the "humoral theory," who maintained that humoral factors alone account for immunity. Each group was confident that its own concept was correct and was unable to perceive that both of these agencies, and others as well, can interact to constitute the total immune response.

Metchnikoff (1905) concluded that "there is only one constant element in immunity, whether innate or acquired, and that is phagocytosis . . . phagocytes . . . ingest micro-organisms and absorb soluble substances . . . seize microbes whilst these are still living . . . and bring them under the action of their cellular contents, which are capable of killing and digesting the micro-organisms or of inhibiting their pathogenic action. Phagocytes act because they possess vital properties and a faculty for exerting a fermentative action on morbific agents. The mechanism of this action is not definitely settled, and we can foresee that for future researches there will be a vast and fertile field to be reached by pursuing this path."

Over half a century later most of these statements are still apropos, and have been confirmed by a tremendous amount of data which has accumulated during the interim, largely as the result of advances in techniques. For example, electron microscopy has permitted study of the ultrastructure of cells, the ultracentrifuge has allowed separation and characterization of cellular components, and the development of radioactive-labeling techniques has provided a tool for studying the sources and metabolism of various cell types.

Subsequent chapters are devoted to some of the most important evidence pertaining to the sources and characteristics of macrophages. Limitations of space do not permit a complete review of the vast literature on these subjects. However, the references listed offer additional information on the topics discussed.

Metchnikoff was, indeed, correct when he foresaw a "vast and fertile field" of research into the activities of macrophages. The works presently discussed give further insight into the scope of this field and afford indications of the large amount of investigation that remains to be done.

SUMMARY: The macrophage is defined as a ubiquitous large mononuclear cell type, capable of phagocytizing particulates and of storing vital dyes. Some of the basic contributions of Metchnikoff, which led to an appreciation of the importance of the macrophage and gave indications of the mechanisms of its activity, are discussed. The perspicacity of Metchnikoff's observations pointed the way to much of the subsequent work in this field, which has been greatly facilitated by technological advances. In subsequent chapters, information will be presented concerning macrophage sources and characteristics.

Chapter 2
The Structure of Macrophages

MACROPHAGES are found in all organs of the mammalian body. When the marked differences in environment within various organs are considered, the finding that the morphology of these cells varies according to their location is not unexpected. Moreover, the morphology of macrophages varies depending on their state of activity.

A. Monocytes

A classical description of monocytes, seen in stained smears of peripheral blood examined with light microscopy, was presented by Bloom (1938a). The blood monocyte, which normally constitutes 3 to 8% of the circulating leukocytes, is a spherical cell as large or larger than the granulocyte, approximately 10 to 11 μ in diameter. Its rounded nucleus is usually indented, and the cell contains a more abundant cytoplasm than do lymphocytes. The characteristics of the monocyte nucleus are thought to reflect the state of maturity of the cell, an elongated nucleus with peripherally distributed clumped chromatin being found in more mature cells. The cytoplasm is slightly basophilic and is often finely reticulated. It has numerous vacuoles and may contain many small azurophilic granules.

Living monocytes observed with phase microscopy frequently exhibit a finely granular cytoplasm resembling "ground glass," in contrast to the more refractile homogeneous cytoplasm of lymphocytes. Supravital staining with Janus green reveals the presence of a large number of short rodlike mitochondria, which frequently occur in a group near the centrosphere. With neutral red supravital staining, a rosette of neutral red vacuoles is often seen in the cytoplasm near the nuclear indentation. The Golgi apparatus also is found in this region.

Bessis (1956), by use of phase microscopy, demonstrated that monocytes move in the same manner as tissue macrophages. The cell assumes a triangular shape, with one angle pointing towards the rear and a hyaloplasmic veil along the advancing margin. The undulating cytoplasmic veil is extremely active under appropriate conditions, as can be seen by cinematography. Phase contrast microscopy also reveals granules, vacuoles, and

5

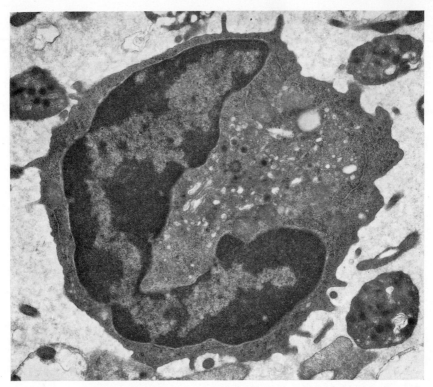

FIGURE 2-1. Electron micrograph of a normal blood monocyte from a guinea pig. Magnification: 12,865. (Courtesy of David Simpson and Russell Ross.)

rod-shaped mitochondria in an abundant light-gray cytoplasm, and one or two nucleoli may be seen in the nucleus. The cells have a distinct tendency to adhere to and spread on glass (Forteza, 1964).

Electron microscopy (EM) has served to emphasize certain character- istics of blood monocytes which aid in distinguishing them from large lymphocytes (Low and Freeman, 1958). Monocytes contain numerous small circular or rod-shaped mitochondria, many small round or oval profiles of endoplasmic reticulum (ER), and some ribosomes in an abun- dant cytoplasm. Lymphocytes, on the other hand, contain but few mito- chondria, little ER, and few ribosomes in a sparse cytoplasm. Differences between the nuclei of monocytes and lymphocytes, as seen by EM, are particularly striking. Monocytes have a characteristic dark, irregular band of chromatin adjacent to the inner margin of the nuclear membrane, while the chromatin of lymphocytes is regularly dispersed throughout the nucleus.

B. *Peritoneal Macrophages*

Peritoneal macrophages are easily obtained from experimental animals and hence have been studied more extensively than other macrophages. In

Giemsa-stained or May-Grünwald-Giemsa-stained preparations examined by light microscopy, peritoneal macrophages frequently measure 10 to 30 μ in diameter, and have nuclei approximately 6 to 12 μ in diameter. The abundant cytoplasm is slightly basophilic, may contain many vacuoles and granules, and gives evidence of being actively ameboid. The eccentric nucleus is oval or kidney-shaped and stains more lightly than the nucleus of a lymphocyte (Maximow, 1924; 1932).

By phase contrast microscopy, peritoneal macrophages are seen to contain abundant light-gray diffuse cytoplasm with darker-gray rod-shaped mitochondria frequently grouped near the centrosphere. Granules and vacuoles occur in the cytoplasm in varying numbers depending on the physiological state of the cell. The pronounced tendency of macrophages to adhere to and spread on glass surfaces creates hyaloplasmic flow which gives rise to expansions of the characteristic veil-like undulating membrane (Policard, 1957).

North and Mackaness (1963a) examined peritoneal macrophages with the electron microscope. Normal peritoneal macrophages from nonimmunized mice were shown to have characteristics which are typical of the peritoneal macrophages of many species. The cytoplasm is enclosed by a three-layered unit membrane, approximately 80 Å thick, with many protuberances and invaginations indicating a high degree of activity. Peripheral cytoplasm in the numerous cellular processes is finely granular and

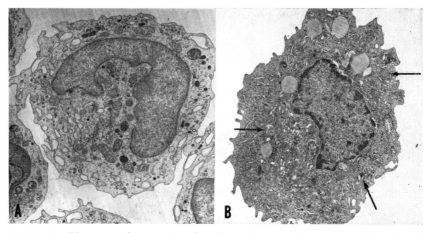

FIGURE 2-2. Electron micrographs of peritoneal macrophages. A, Nonactivated macrophage washed directly from the peritoneum of a germ-free rat, without an inducer of exudate. The cytoplasm contains relatively few ribosomes and electron-dense lysosomes. Magnification: 5,060. B, Activated macrophage washed from the peritoneum of a rabbit 4 days after the injection of Bayol F. The nuclear material is aggregated adjacent to the nuclear membrane. The cytoplasm contains innumerable ribosomes, a substantial amount of rough endoplasmic reticulum, large phagosomes filled with the injected oil, and many small lysosomes and phagolysosomes (arrows). Magnification: 5,060. (Courtesy of E. S. Leake and Q. N. Myrvik.)

usually lacks the structures seen in the rest of the cytoplasm, i.e. membranes of ER with and without attached ribosomes, many free ribosomes approximately 30 Å in diameter often arranged in polysomes, and cylindrical mitochondria 0.3 to 0.5 μ in diameter and 1.5 to 2.0 μ long. Cytoplasmic vesicles 300 Å to 0.5 μ in diameter, enclosed by a unit membrane, are of three main types: small pinocytic vesicles, various-sized organelles containing a fine granular material, and larger, denser vacuoles. The nucleus is oval with one or more indentations and is enclosed by a porous double-unit membrane. Nucleoli are sometimes seen. Ribosomes are attached to the external portion of the nuclear membrane, which appears to be continuous with the ER. The centrosome, opposite the nuclear indentation, is a spherical region of about 5 cu μ of finely granular cytoplasm containing one or more fibrous centrioles and is surrounded by groups of Golgi membranes. Many investigators have reported similar observations on the ultrastructure of mouse peritoneal macrophages (e.g. Carr, 1967).

Stimuli of various kinds, such as those which accompany the phagocytosis of bacteria, can cause "macrophage activation." An "activated macrophage" is one which is metabolically highly active and contains many organelles, including lysosomes rich in hydrolytic enzymes. Following ingestion of *Listeria monocytogenes* by mouse peritoneal macrophages, North and Mackaness (1963a) observed the bacteria within phagocytic vacuoles (phagosomes), surrounded at first by a clear area bounded by a unit membrane. Later, the clear area was filled with an amorphous material which apparently had been transferred from cytoplasmic vesicles (lysosomes) into the phagosomes to form phagolysosomes.

The peritoneal macrophages of mice that have survived an initial infection with *L. monocytogenes* are regarded to be "immune" since they can kill the specific organism rather than support its intracellular growth. North and Mackaness (1963b) compared the ultrastructure of peritoneal macrophages from mice immunized with *L. monocytogenes* with that of peritoneal macrophages from nonimmunized mice. The cytoplasmic membrane of immune macrophages is smoother, and has fewer protuberances and invaginations than the membrane of nonimmunized macrophages. There are many free ribosomes but very few profiles of ER. The mitochondria are smaller, more numerous and contain more cristae. Compared with nonimmune peritoneal macrophages the cytoplasm of immune macrophages is less dense and appears to be highly hydrated. It contains fewer vesicles and a very extensive Golgi apparatus. Nucleoli are usually seen within the nucleus. It was suggested that these differences between immune and nonimmune cells probably result from the emergence in immune mice of a new population of peritoneal macrophages which are in the process of differentiation.

Peritoneal macrophages from nonimmunized hamsters are similar to those of the mouse described above, as evidenced by the EM studies of

Dumont and Sheldon (1965). The mitochondria of hamster peritoneal macrophages were rounded, the rough ER was sparse, and nuclei showed areas of electron-dense chromatin adjacent to the inner margin of the nuclear membrane. Ultrastructural changes of great interest were also seen within macrophages containing tubercle bacilli. The ingested bacilli were seen in clear, empty phagosomes, which became surrounded by lysosomes that fused to engulf the whole phagosome. Subsequently the phagosomal membrane disappeared and the tubercle bacilli appeared to be in direct contact with the electron-dense lysosomal material. In other instances, phagosomes containing bacilli became permeated by vesicles containing low-density material; concentric rings of granular substance developed around the bacilli and finally transformed into calcified bodies. A loss of density of the cytoplasm of macrophages in the lesion was correlated with the appearance of epithelioid cells observed by light microscopy.

Mouse and hamster peritoneal macrophages are not appreciably different in morphology from other mammalian and avian peritoneal macrophages, e.g. rat and chicken (Palade, 1955); rabbit (Casley-Smith and Day, 1966) or guinea pig (Karlsbad et al., 1964).

C. Alveolar Macrophages

The structure of alveolar macrophages of various species of animals is similar and differs from that of macrophages from other locations, presumably because of unique features of the pulmonary environment other than heavy exposure to foreign particulates. The morphology of alveolar macrophages from germ-free and conventionally reared animals is essentially the same (Bauer, 1968). Leake and Heise (1967) have summarized evidence, obtained by electron and light microscopy, which supports the concept that alveolar and peritoneal macrophages represent two morphologically distinct cell types. They observed five major morphological differences between alveolar and peritoneal macrophages of germ-free rats. First, the nuclei of alveolar macrophages are rounded or slightly ovoid and nucleoli are seen more often than in peritoneal macrophages. The latter characteristically have elongated, deeply-indented nuclei. Second, rough ER is seen frequently in peritoneal, but rarely in alveolar, macrophages. Third, peritoneal macrophages have a more extensive Golgi apparatus than do alveolar macrophages. Fourth, alveolar macrophages have many dense cytoplasmic granules which are not observed in peritoneal macrophages. Fifth, the mitochondria in peritoneal macrophages are larger and more elongated than mitochondria of alveolar macrophages. In addition, the overall diameter of the alveolar macrophage is approximately 1.5 times that of the peritoneal macrophage. $9\mu - 18\mu$

Kajita et al. (1959) studied the alveolar macrophages of soot-exposed mice with the electron microscope. The inhaled soot particles were com-

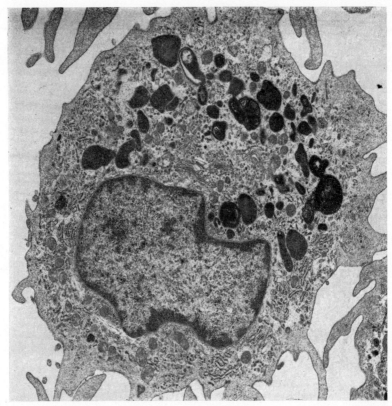

FIGURE 2-3. Electron micrograph of a naturally activated alveolar macrophage from a nonimmunized rabbit. The cell appears to be moderately active, as evidenced by the clumped nuclear material adjacent to the nuclear membrane, a well-developed Golgi apparatus, and a moderate number of ribosomes, phagosomes, and phagolysosomes. Phagocytized material can be seen within many of the phagolysosomes. Magnification: 9,200. (Courtesy of E. S. Leake and Q. N. Myrvik.)

monly seen within clear membrane-bound vacuoles. The cells contained eccentric rounded nuclei in an abundant low-density cytoplasm, and had a high cytoplasm-to-nucleus ratio. Their mitochondria were elongated with regularly arranged cristae and the cell membranes presented many processes and invaginations. Karrer (1958; 1960) reported similar observations on the morphology of normal mouse alveolar macrophages and those that had phagocytized India ink.

Moore and Schoenberg (1964) examined the alveolar macrophages of rabbits. Policard et al. (1957) studied alveolar cells from a variety of higher animals and Nagaishi et al. (1964) compared the lung morphology of mammals with that of lower animals. It is evident from the reports of these investigators that the ultrastructure of normal alveolar macrophages of the various higher animals is similar.

D. *Splenic Macrophages*

Palade (1956) described rat splenic macrophages, which are ultrastructurally similar to peritoneal macrophages. The specialized activities of splenic macrophages, i.e. removal of large proportions of effete cells, are reflected in their structure. Swartzendruber and Congdon (1963) and Swartzendruber (1964; 1967) reported EM observations on mouse spleen tingible-body macrophages which had phagocytized cellular debris, possibly derived from small lymphocytes or erythrocytes; phagocytized plasma cells were clearly identifiable within the macrophages. These splenic macrophages were 20 to 30 μ or larger in diameter, with nuclei measuring 12 to 15 μ. The nuclei were typical of macrophages in the peritoneum and elsewhere, with chromatin peripherally located. Usually two dense nucleoli were present. The cells contained smooth and rough ER and a well-developed Golgi apparatus.

E. *Macrophages of Lymph Nodes and Thymus*

Lymph nodes contain various kinds of macrophages. The electron micrographs of Ada *et al.* (1967) show typical macrophages lining the medullary sinuses of lymph nodes, and characteristic tingible-body macrophages in the germinal centers of secondary follicles in the cortex. Ada *et al.* also described reticular cells with long, dendritic processes, which are capable of retaining antigen on their surfaces. These cells have certain characteristics of macrophages. Although they are not actively phagocytic, they can store dye and have the capacity to phagocytize materials under certain circumstances. Thus, they apparently represent inactive macrophages.

Fresen (1960) described the ramifying, thin cytoplasmic processes of lymph node reticular cells, which are similar in appearance to Kupffer cells. Braunstein *et al.* (1958) studied macrophages of human lymph nodes, using hematoxylin and eosin-stained or special histochemically stained sections. These stellate cells had reniform nuclei, many ramifying processes, and measured 20 to 40 μ overall.

Germinal centers in tonsils from patients with chronic tonsillitis were described by Lennert, Caesar, and Müller (1967). The macrophages in the reticulum of these lymphoid tissues had nuclei with clumped chromatin and a dense central nucleolus, smooth ER but few ribosomes, many cytoplasmic inclusions, and numerous cytoplasmic extensions. Portions of ingested cells were commonly seen in these activated macrophages, either as tingible bodies, identifiable cell remnants, or myelin figures.

A study of the ultrastructure of mouse lymph nodes after skin grafting has revealed the presence of increased numbers of macrophages by 24 hours after grafting (Simar, Betz, and Lejeune, 1967). Macrophages in lymph node sinuses contained much cytoplasm and a considerable amount of phagocytized material, including osmiophilic granules.

Macrophages of the thymus resemble those of lymph nodes in structure (Clark, 1963). Kostowiecki (1963) extensively reviewed the literature on thymic macrophages.

F. Liver Macrophages (Kupffer Cells)

Kupffer cells constitute approximately 30% of the nucleated cells of the liver! Various methods have been described for separating them from liver parenchymal cells (e.g. St. George, 1960; Garvey, 1961; Bennett, 1966; Pisano, Filkins, and DiLuzio, 1967; Mills and Zucker-Franklin, 1969). Many years ago, Rous and Beard (1934) described a method for separating Kupffer cells from nonphagocytic cells in liver perfusate. The macrophages were allowed to ingest minute particles of iron prior to liver perfusion and were subsequently removed from suspension with a magnet. Beard and Rous (1934) cultivated the isolated Kupffer cells *in vitro* and characterized them. They recognized morphological similarities between liver macrophages and macrophages from other sources and grouped all of these cells together as members of the reticuloendothelial system. They also stressed that certain differences exist between fixed Kupffer cells and free macrophages of exudates or macrophages of the spleen and other organs. For example, they reported that the surfaces of Kupffer cells are considerably stickier than those of other macrophages and hence these cells are difficult to handle *in vitro*. It was their opinion that Kupffer cells are easily distinguishable from other macrophages.

Kupffer cells were visualized by EM in the investigations of deMan *et al.* (1960), who reported that these irregularly shaped cells project into the lumen of the sinuses that they line and have fine cytoplasmic extensions inserted between adjacent parenchymal cells. The surface area of the cells is large because of the many projections and invaginations of these cells. Portal blood flows directly through the liver sinuses and over the large surface area of the Kupffer cells, providing them with the opportunity to adsorb and dispose of substances from the gastrointestinal tract. The cytoplasm of these cells contains many mitochondria and electron-dense bodies, which deMan *et al.* (1960) called cytosomes; however, these enzyme-rich bodies probably represented lysosomes and phagolysosomes. The intensive phagocytic activities of Kupffer cells are reflected in the EM observations made by Rouiller (1962), who found that they contain many vesicles, lysosomes, phagosomes, and some erythrocytes in various stages of digestion.

Matter and co-workers (1968) made a stereological analysis of the fine structure of the "micropinocytosis vermiformis" in Kupffer cells of the rat. This structure, said to be characteristic of all macrophages, is made up of tubular and lamellar portions, usually parallel to the cell surface, which join to form an intricate labyrinth. About one tenth of the tubular structures communicate with the pinocytic system; the rest form a dense layer around the pinocytic system, which communicates with the extracellular environment. This "micropinocytosis vermiformis" affords a means of facilitating the entrance of materials into the cell.

G. Central Nervous System Macrophages (Microglia Cells)

Microglia cells (Hortega cells, mesoglia) have long been considered to be macrophages, since in conditions of trauma they become typical ameboid phagocytic cells (Truex, 1959). Under normal conditions, resting microglia cells do not store intravenously injected dyes because the wall of astroglia surrounding blood vessels prevents dye from reaching them. If the wall is injured to allow dye penetration, it can be shown that microglia cells will store dyes. Hortega cells which have lost their processes and have transformed to free macrophages have been called "compound granular corpuscles," Gitterzellen, or lipophages. Gitterzellen are very similar in appearance to Kupffer cells (Jaffé, 1938).

Hosokawa and Mannen (1963) and Honjin (1963) studied neuroglia cells by light and electron microscopy and tabulated the characteristics of the different types. They reported that microglia cells are found in both gray and white matter. The average cell length for human resting microglia is 61.6 μ, for monkey 52.2 μ, and for rabbit 53.2 μ, with respective nuclear lengths of 12.6 μ, 10.6 μ, and 8.1 μ. The chromatin-rich nucleus is irregular or twisted in shape and presents one nucleolus. The cytoplasm contains a moderate number of mitochondria, many vacuoles and granules, a large amount of ER, and clumps of Golgi membranes.

Resting microglia cells have a rod-shaped or triangular nucleus with very thin, branching, spiny cytoplasmic processes. The bipolar microglial cell is called a "rod cell" because the nucleus assumes an elongated rod form between two thin bipolar cytoplasmic processes, which may be branched at each end. Other forms with angular nuclei have three, four, or occasionally more processes arising from the angles around the nucleus and are called tripolar, quadripolar, or multipolar respectively.

Microglia cells may be perineuronal or perivascular satellites, with spiny processes attached to either a nerve cell or blood vessel or connecting the two. The reasons for these cell associations are not known, since the microglia cells do not usually form foot processes, as do the astroglia cells which contribute to the blood-brain barrier.

As previously stated, following trauma the thin spiny processes of resting microglia cells are lost, the cytoplasm swells, and the cells resemble free macrophages found at other loci in the body.

H. Macrophages of Other Organs and Tissues

In addition to macrophages of blood, peritoneum, lungs, spleen, lymph nodes, liver, and the central nervous system, macrophages are present in virtually every other organ and tissue. They are ultrastructurally similar, except for lung macrophages, although, as shown above, the environment and state of activity of the cell may be reflected by alterations in morphology.

Although the morphology of macrophages of organs other than those listed above will not be discussed separately, the following references are pertinent. Salm (1962) described the activities of phagocytic mononuclear cells in lesions of the uterus; Bulmer (1964) described rat ovarian macrophages; Phadke and Phadke (1961) and Carr *et al.* (1968) reported on macrophages in normal and abnormal conditions in male reproductive organs; Mayberry (1964) observed macrophages in post-secretory mammary involution; Berman (1967) presented excellent descriptions of macrophages in bone marrow; and Niebauer (1968) described the melanophage or macrophage of the skin.

I. *Epithelioid Cells and Giant Cells*

Although Metchnikoff (1888) described the presence of epithelioid and giant cells in tuberculous lesions, much remains to be learned about these cell types. There is general agreement that they are reticulohistiocytic cells. In certain diseases, including tuberculosis, sarcoidosis, and silicosis, they are found in lymph nodes as well as in granulomatous lesions. Rich (1951a) discussed the factors responsible for the formation of epithelioid and giant cells and described their appearance. During transformation to the epithelioid cell, the macrophage is highly activated and its nucleus increases in size. At least two types of giant cells are found in granulomas. The Langhans' giant cell has multiple nuclei located at its periphery, while the foreign-body giant cell contains numerous centrally located nuclei.

Maturation of macrophages to epithelioid and giant cells in hamsters given killed tubercle bacilli was described by Dumont and Sheldon (1965). Giant cells and early epithelioid cells derived from mature macrophages had electron-dense cytoplasm, which became less dense as the cells aged.

Sutton and Weiss (1966) described chick epithelioid cells which had developed from monocytes *in vitro*. Electron microscopy revealed polygonal cells with an epithelial appearance, containing a nucleus with finely dispersed chromatin, two or more nucleoli, and numerous nuclear pores. The cytoplasm was rich in organelles, including free ribosomes and polysomes, mitochondria, and lysosomes. Prominent cuplike structures in the cytoplasmic membrane were thought to be remnants of lysosomes which had discharged their contents extracellularly. Mitochondria were more numerous and larger than in the less mature monocytes and the macrophages which preceded the epithelioid cells. The mitochondria were as long as 2.0 μ and appeared to be dilated. Isolated profiles of rough ER were present and many lysosomes of varying sizes and densities were seen. Many filaments 50 to 60 Å in diameter or larger, frequently in bundles,

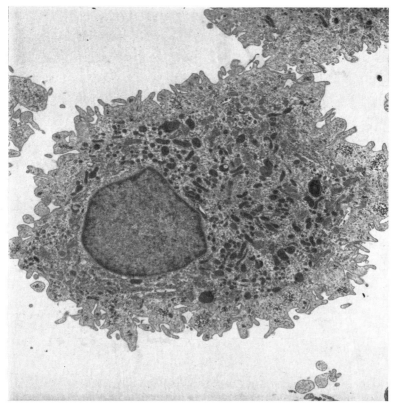

FIGURE 2-4. Electron micrograph of an epithelioid cell obtained from the lungs of a rabbit injected intratracheally with living *Mycobacterium smegmatis* 5 days before the micrograph was taken. The nucleus appears rounded and shows some margination of chromatin; the cytoplasm contains a large number of electron-dense lysosomes, bearing evidence of extensive cellular activity. Magnification: 5,500. (Courtesy of E. S. Leake and Q. N. Myrvik.)

were present in the cytoplasm. The cells did not contain intact phagosomes, but large, clear vacuoles were interpreted to be remnants of phagosomes and phagolysosomes. These epithelioid cells sometimes contained a "remarkable structure" consisting of concentric rows of small vesicles similar to those in the Golgi region, but located in the peripheral cytoplasm. It is possible that this structure represents a "pinocytic apparatus," similar to that described by Matter *et al.* (1968).

In this *in vitro* study, Sutton and Weiss (1966) also examined giant cells. Their large masses of cytoplasm contained large, clear cytoplasmic vacuoles and as many as 150 nuclei were present. Many characteristics of the cells were similar to those of the epithelioid cell; however, lysosomes were absent.

The macrophages of granulomas of rats fuse to form giant cells. Labeling studies of Silverman and Shorter (1963) gave no evidence for division of nuclei following cell fusion. However, this question remains unsettled.

SUMMARY: Macrophages are found throughout the mammalian body. Those found in many locations are similar in morphology. However, alveolar macrophages exhibit striking structural differences from most other macrophages, presumably due to the uniqueness of the lung environment; they are easily distinguished by virtue of their smooth oval nucleus and high cytoplasm-to-nucleus ratio.

In general, macrophages have eccentrically located, indented, reniform nuclei, frequently with peripheral chromatin and one or two nucleoli. In activated macrophages the cytoplasm is abundant and contains many vesicles, including lysosomes, phagosomes, and phagolysosomes. Epithelioid and giant cells apparently are terminal forms of macrophages which give morphological evidence of having been extremely active. Epithelioid cells contain lysosomes but no intact phagosomes, and giant cells often lack both lysosomes and intact phagocytic vacuoles.

Chapter 3

The Phylogeny and
Ontogeny of Macrophages

A. *Phylogeny*

Macrophages of various animal species were studied extensively by Metchnikoff (1905), whose descriptions of the digestion of red blood cells (RBCs) by macrophages in the flatworm are highly graphic. When the worms were fed goose RBCs the nuclei and hemoglobin made it possible to trace the fate of the ingested cells. Phagocytic cells in the worm intestinal epithelium rapidly ingested the RBCs, and subsequently digested them slowly but completely. In the Coelenterata, intracellular digestion could be observed directly *in vivo,* since these animals are transparent. The actinians, or sea-anemones, also proved to be good subjects for study. These animals eat many types of food, including shrimp. The empty shrimp shells are ejected and particles of the meat are engulfed and digested by phagocytic cells in the intestinal epithelium, in a manner similar to that observed in the flatworm. Since these phagocytes can also take up neutral red and other dyes, they are classified as macrophages. Metchnikoff presented evidence supporting the concept that these cells are entirely responsible for the primitive digestion of lower animals. With increasing phylogenetic complexity, this primitive digestive function carried out by phagocytes is replaced by enzymes secreted by specialized cells of the alimentary system. The macrophages of higher animals, however, retain some digestive capabilities, which aid in tissue resorption and other functions.

The reticuloendothelial apparatus of a complex and highly developed invertebrate, the lesser octopus *Eledone cirrosa,* has been studied by Stuart (1968). This octopus lacks lymphatics and discrete foci of lymphoid tissue, but has a "white body" which serves as the leukoformative organ. Carbon particles injected into the octopus were observed to localize within large collections of phagocytic cells in the gill and the post-salivary gland, and in some phagocytes of the "white body." A single type of ameboid cell was found in the blood. It resembled typical macrophages seen in other animals, and was cultured *in vitro* for periods of up to 4 days. Although the blood lacked agglutinins for bacteria, yeast, or RBCs, it contained opsonins (presumably nonspecific) for these particles, which greatly facilitated their phagocytosis by macrophages.

Metchnikoff also described polymorphonuclear neutrophils (PMNs) and macrophages in many higher animals, including mammals, the *Alligator mississipiensis,* and even one of the lowest vertebrate forms, the lamprey. Although PMNs of all these species can ingest foreign erythrocytes, macrophages show stronger positive chemotaxis toward foreign RBCs and are chiefly responsible for their destruction.

Antibacterial cellular immunity can be demonstrated easily in various species of fish, as shown by Mesnil (1895). Perch, gudgeon, and goldfish resisted intraperitoneal infection with *Bacillus anthracis* despite the fact that their peritoneal fluids readily supported growth of the bacilli *in vitro* at temperatures of 15 to 23° C. Mesnil clearly showed that the macrophages of osseous fishes are responsible for immunity to this organism even though it remains within the macrophages for long periods before being killed.

The temperature dependence of both phagocytosis and cellular immunity in various species was reviewed by Mesnil (1895), Metchnikoff (1905), and later by Bisset (1946, 1947).

Berry and Spies (1949) reviewed the literature on phagocytosis in certain lower animals, including invertebrates.

In recent studies on antigen clearance from the circulation by the macrophages of various species, Nelstrop, Taylor, and Collard (1968a, b, c) found that clearance of a second dose of T_1 bacteriophage was more rapid than clearance of a primary dose of the phage in the goldfish, lamprey, and shore crab, but not in the dogfish or land snail. They concluded that an immune response, phylogenetically more primitive than that concerned with humoral antibody formation, may exist in these animals. Apparently this postulated primitive response is concerned with a macrophage-associated cellular immunity, and is nonspecific. However, the possibility that macrophages of fishes may participate in specific immune reactions is suggested by the finding of Chiller *et al.* (1969) that macrophages from fish immunized with sheep RBCs can form rosettes, evidently because of surface cytophilic antibodies.

It is obvious that various activities of macrophages contribute to body economy throughout a wide spectrum of the phylogenetic scale.

B. Ontogeny

The origin and development of the reticuloendothelial system (RES) in human embryos was described by Richter (1958), who also reviewed much of the earlier literature on this subject.

The ontogeny of the macrophage in human fetal tissues has been well described by Andersen and Matthiessen (1966), who reported that macrophages of typical morphology are widespread in fetal tissues. These cells exhibit ameboid motility, and have marked pinocytic and phagocytic capabilities. Their lysosomes contain an abundance of acid hydrolytic enzymes and fuse with phagosomes in characteristic fashion to form phagolysosomes. The cells appear to digest tissue, especially in certain areas undergoing embryonic development. In the early fetus they are found both within vessels and in perivascular connective tissue, but never in nonvascular mesenchyme. For this reason, Andersen and Matthiessen contend that these cells originate from "primitive leukocytes." Apparently they can differentiate into chondroclasts and multinucleated osteoclasts, as well as microglia cells.

The functional development of the RES in animal fetuses has been the subject of recent investigation. The phagocytic capacity of the RES develops progressively during fetal life of the rat (Reade and Jenkin, 1965) and the chick (Karthigasu and Jenkin, 1963), but fails to reach adult levels by the time of birth. Histological studies (Reade and Casley-Smith, 1965) revealed that Kupffer cells are capable of taking up intravenously injected particles from the circulation of fetal rats at the earliest time studied, 14 days after conception; however, their phagocytic efficiency increased with increasing age of the fetus. Karthigasu, Reade, and Jenkin (1965) examined the antibacterial capacity of fixed macrophages of both rats and chicks. They demonstrated that, even in the presence of specific antibodies, fetal macrophages generally lack the capacity to kill certain gram-negative bacteria following phagocytosis. It is probable that this attribute develops soon after birth, because the macrophages of neonatal animals were observed to possess bactericidal capabilities. However, the macrophages of adults are more active than those of newborn animals (Reade, 1968).

Certain components of C', known to be synthesized by macrophages of adult animals (see Chapter 6), are also synthesized by the human fetus (Propp and Alper, 1968). Adinolfi, Gardner, and Wood (1968) demonstrated that macrophage-rich tissues, such as liver, lung, and peritoneal cells, taken from fetuses 10 weeks of age or older synthesize β_{1C-1A} globulins *in vitro*. Tissues from 14-week-old fetuses made β_{1E} globulin as well. These findings make it reasonably certain that macrophages acquire some of their specialized synthetic capabilities early in ontogeny.

SUMMARY: Macrophages are found in all animals. In the most primitive invertebrates they are totally responsible for the digestion of food and the disposal of foreign materials. In higher animals, some of their primitive digestive activities are replaced by enzymes secreted by other cells; however, macrophages retain digestive capabilities which aid in tissue resorption and other functions.

Antibacterial cellular immunity is a characteristic function of macrophages throughout a wide phylogenetic range. Whereas, in the lower animals, a primitive nonspecific response results in a macrophage-associated

cellular immunity, most of the vertebrate species can apparently supplement this by providing for specific immune activities of macrophages,
through the agency of cytophilic antibodies or other means.

During the ontogeny of mammals, macrophages appear early and are
active in resorption of tissue during embryonic development. They acquire
many of their synthetic capabilities very early during ontogeny, as evidenced
by their ability to synthesize hydrolytic enzymes and certain components
of complement. The phagocytic capabilities of the RES increase progressively during fetal and neonatal life.

Chapter 4

Sources, Maturation, and Life Span of Macrophages

THE SOURCES, maturation, and life span of macrophages have been subjects of much conjecture. For many years, light microscopy was virtually the only tool available for studying these problems; in recent years, techniques for radioactive labeling and tracing of cell division and migration have provided better approaches.

A. Bone Marrow Stem Cells as Progenitors of Macrophages

Experiments using radiation chimeras have provided evidence that the bone marrow is a major source of macrophage precursors. Indeed it has been suggested that bone marrow stem cells serve as the sole primary origin of macrophages (Virolainen and Defendi, 1968). Balner (1963) transplanted mouse bone marrow cells into lethally x-irradiated recipients. Cytotoxicity tests conducted with specific alloantisera demonstrated that at 6 weeks all of the free peritoneal macrophages in the resulting chimeras were derived from the transferred bone marrow cells. In similar experiments, Goodman (1964) showed that at various times, ranging from several months to over a year after transfer of bone marrow, virtually all of the peritoneal macrophages in the recipients were of donor origin.

Other experimental evidence likewise strongly supports the thesis that cells from the bone marrow serve as the principal progenitors of macrophages. For example, parabiosis experiments have demonstrated conclusively that many exudative macrophages are derived from blood-borne cells (Volkman and Gowans, 1965a). The common circulation between two parabiosed rats was interrupted long enough to label cells in one of the partners with a pulse of tritiated thymidine. Subsequent radioautography showed that a substantial number of macrophages in induced inflammatory exudates of the unlabeled partner were labeled, and hence were blood-borne, presumably monocytes from bone marrow. Studies with labeled cells further indicated that precursors of macrophages proliferate rapidly and continuously in areas distant from the inflammatory site, and release their progeny into the circulation. The extent and characteristics of labeling of peritoneal exudate cells in rats given tritiated thymidine also indicated that a population of morphologically unidentified bone marrow cells provides precursors of peritoneal macrophages (Volkman, 1966). In addition, histochemical staining indicates that certain cells in bone marrow serve as precursors of monocytes and that there is a continuous flow of monocytes from the marrow (Braunsteiner and Schmalzl, 1968).

Still other evidence which supports the concept that bone marrow cells serve as principal progenitors of macrophages, as well as other cells, found in inflammatory lesions has come from the work of Spector and Willoughby (1968). These investigators transfused lymph node, thymus, or bone marrow cells into rats treated with 600 r of x-irradiation. It was found that, whereas rats restored with lymph node or thymus cells lacked the capacity to mount a cellular inflammatory response, animals which received bone marrow cells regained this capacity.

Macrophages in other locations have also been shown to be derived from cells in the bone marrow. Pinkett, Cowdrey, and Nowell (1966) used mice made chimeric by the transfer of marrow cells carrying the T_6 chromosome marker into syngeneic x-irradiated mice. Approximately two thirds of the alveolar macrophages arose from the transfused cells; evidently the remaining one third were derived from existing pulmonary tissue. It has been conclusively shown that macrophages in the liver normally develop mainly from bone marrow precursors, as reviewed by Boak et al. (1968).

B. Blood Monocytes as Circulating Immature Macrophages

There is general agreement that blood monocytes can mature into tissue and exudative macrophages (Ebert and Florey, 1939; Tompkins, 1955; Lawkowicz and Krzeminska-Lawkowicz, 1957; Rebuck and LoGrippo, 1961; Spector, Walters, and Willoughby, 1965; Spector and Coote, 1965; Hurd and Ziff, 1968).

The recent radioautographic studies of Volkman and Gowans (1965a), Trepel and Begemann (1966), and Gillman and Wright (1966) have suggested that blood monocytes account for many of the macrophages in local inflammatory sites.

The importance of environmental stimuli in the differentiation of macrophages was stressed by Carrel and Ebeling (1926a, b) and Carrel (1934) many years ago. These investigators concluded that macrophages merely represent highly differentiated monocytes. Furthermore, they showed that differentiation can occur in vitro and depends on the medium used. Transformation of mouse monocytes into typical macrophages was observed in vitro and in vivo by Cohn and Benson (1965a).

The in vitro transformation of chicken monocytes into macrophages, then into epithelioid cells, and finally into multinucleated giant cells was described by Lewis (1925) and by Hetherington and Pierce (1931). Sutton and Weiss (1966) studied leukocyte cultures of cardiac blood of chickens by light and electron microscopy. The most active phagocytosis of particulates by mononuclear cells occurred between 6 and 24 hours. After one day in culture a monolayer of macrophages developed. Many of these cells transformed into epithelioid cells between days 3 and 6. Giant cells appeared as early as 2 to 4 days and were commonly present at 9 to 15 days.

That human monocytes readily transform into macrophages *in vitro* was shown by Lewis (1925) and by Berman and Stulberg (1962). The work of Rabinowitz and Schrek (1962) is particularly informative. These investigators used phase microscopy and cinemicrography to follow the transformation of human blood monocytes into mature macrophages; the transformation occurred in about one week.

Bennett and Cohn (1966) obtained relatively pure suspensions of monocytes from horse blood by flotation on dense albumin solutions. Further purification was achieved by allowing the monocytes to adhere to the culture vessel at 37° C for 2 hours, at which time most of the contaminating lymphocytes were washed away. Culture for 24 to 72 hours resulted in transformation of the monocytes into typical activated macrophages, as evidenced by their functional and biochemical characteristics. The authors, in agreement with van Furth and Cohn (1968), suggested that the probable development of macrophages from monocytes *in vivo* is as follows: blood monocytes are derived from the bone marrow and have a short half-life in the circulation before emigrating through capillaries into tissues, particularly in response to inflammatory stimuli; within tissues they mature to become typical macrophages.

C. *Other Possible Sources of Macrophages*

In addition to bone marrow stem cells and peripheral blood monocytes, mature macrophages arise from other precursors. The possible transformation of lymphocytes to macrophages will be discussed in Section D of this chapter.

Early investigators believed that endothelial cells could give rise to macrophages. However, Sacks (1926) noted that Aschoff could find no evidence that phagocytes originate from vascular endothelium, but only from "specialized endothelium" in organs such as the liver and spleen. The present consensus is that certain of the cells adhering to endothelium of the sinuses of liver and spleen are inactive macrophages (littoral cells) and not true endothelial cells (Florey, 1962) and that vascular endothelium does not give rise to free phagocytes.

It has also been proposed that tissue mesenchyme is a source of macrophages. Libansky (1966) used the skin-window technique in an attempt to define the source of macrophages at local inflammatory sites in a selected group of patients with various types of leukopenia. Although the intensity of neutrophil infiltration at the skin-window site correlated with the neutrophil count, no correlation was observed between the numbers of mononuclear cells at the site and in the circulation. Even when circulating mononuclear leukocytes were virtually absent the local inflammatory response was normal, provided the blood neutrophil count was normal. It was concluded that the macrophages at sites of inflammation in patients with decreased numbers of circulating mononuclear cells came from tissue mesenchyme. It was further suggested that tissue mesenchyme might serve as a source of macrophages in healthy individuals as well as in leukopenic patients.

Mobilization of histiocytes from tissues and from special organs and structures, such as the "milk spots" of the omentum, is commonly observed. On the basis of studies with the phase microscope, Felix and Dalton (1955) asserted that the majority of macrophages which accumulate in the ascites during inflammation of the peritoneum are mobilized from the omentum and that few, if any, come from the blood stream.

Peritoneal macrophages can proliferate (Felix and Dalton, 1955; Bloom and Fawcett, 1962; Forbes and Mackaness, 1963; Forbes, 1965). Their proliferation results from various stimuli including nonspecific bacterial products (see Chapter 5), antigen (Forbes, 1966), and growth factor produced by fibroblasts (see Chapter 5). Aronson and Elberg (1962) used tritiated thymidine to label the nuclei of rabbit peritoneal macrophages *in vivo* and *in vitro*. They observed that, although macrophages did not divide appreciably during the first 24 hours after injection of an irritant, many labeled cells appeared later suggesting that macrophages had proliferated in the peritoneum.

Virolainen and Defendi (1967) succeeded in inducing division in most of the cells of a macrophage monolayer. Other evidence which indicates that macrophages are capable of division and, furthermore, that they have a life span of weeks or months, has come from the *in vitro* studies of Chang (1964) who claims to have cultivated mouse peritoneal macrophages in good condition for 220 days. Mitotic division occurred early in the course of culture, but the percentage of dividing cells in this *in vitro* system was always less than 0.05%. Bennett (1966, 1967) also reported a low mitotic rate for macrophages *in vitro*. Epstein and Krasnobrod (1968) demonstrated that macrophages divide in experimental granulomas of man and concluded that these cells give rise to the epithelioid cells in the lesions.

Peritoneal macrophages of animals with delayed sensitivity to an antigen are stimulated to divide following contact with the antigen. Whereas only about 1% of peritoneal mononuclear cells from untreated mice synthesized desoxyribose nucleic acid (DNA), Forbes and Mackaness (1963) showed that more than 50% of peritoneal mononuclear cells (predominately macrophages) collected from sensitized animals 20 to 30 hours after challenge with specific antigen were synthesizing DNA. This suggests that division of macrophages mobilized locally is an important source of these cells in exudates associated with delayed sensitivity reactions.

It is conceivable that some of the macrophages associated with delayed sensitivity reactions could be derived from circulating lymphocytes which escape from antigen-stimulated lymph nodes. These lymphocytes are known to be responsible in some way for the development of delayed sensitivity. However, the labeling studies of Turk and Polák (1967) suggest that sensitized lymphocytes from draining lymph nodes do not directly transform or differentiate into macrophages. Turk and Polák found that, 8 days after giving a dose of allergen to produce delayed sensitivity, very few or none of the peritoneal macrophages were derived from cells of the draining lymph nodes.

Although it has been suggested that alveolar macrophages arise from septal cells of the lung (Robertson, 1941), this is only a remote possibility. The septal cells, also known as "great alveolar cells," "type II cells," and "granular pneumocytes," are secretory cells with "cytosomes" presumed to contain surfactant. Sorokin (1966) showed that alveolar macrophages and great alveolar cells differ cytochemically. Great alveolar cells also have limited phagocytic capabilities, as compared with alveolar macrophages. Thus, it is not probable that the two cell types belong to a single cell line.

Mitosis rates of rat alveolar cells were determined by Bertalanffy (1964). The life span of alveolar macrophages, from mitosis to the time of extrusion from the lung, was calculated to be about 27 days or less for the cells with many lipid-containing vacuoles and 9 days for those without large amounts of lipid. These results are essentially in agreement with those of Spencer and Shorter (1962) and Shorter, Titus, and Divertie (1964), who used tritiated-thymidine labeling to determine the turnover time of alveolar cells in mice. These investigators concluded that most alveolar macrophages have a life span of about 7 days, although some labeled cells remained in the lungs for 3 weeks and longer. Similarly, Bowden, Davies, and Wyatt (1968) determined that alveolar macrophages of the mouse have a turnover time of 7 days.

Bertalanffy (1964) reported that most alveolar macrophages are extruded from the respiratory tract into the sputum, and in this manner remove the bulk of inhaled particulate material from the lung. Some alveolar macrophages enter lymph channels, as evidenced by the gross darkening of hilar lymph nodes with accumulated dust particles, especially in older city-dwellers.

The migration of liver macrophages into the lung and their elimination via the respiratory tract has been suggested by the work of Nicol and Cordingly (1966), who found that intravenously injected carbon was stored in Kupffer cells of the rat for several weeks. At 3 to 6 weeks, carbon-laden macrophages, presumably from the liver, appeared in the lungs. Carbon-laden cells in the liver decreased in number over a period of several months, during which time these cells appeared in the lungs. Similar findings were described following trypan blue administration (Nicol and Cordingly, 1967). Nicol and Cordingly suggested that, under normal conditions, some alveolar macrophages may be derived from Kupffer cells and other tissue macrophages. These findings also suggested that macrophages may have a life span of many months. Alternatively, it is possible that the particles were released from the macrophages which originally ingested them, to reach other macrophages. Evidence favoring these possibilities has also been presented by Singer *et al.* (1967) who suggested that this offers a mechanism for recirculation of antigen.

It is difficult, for several reasons, to entertain the concept that in the normal animal an appreciable percent of alveolar macrophages represent migrated Kupffer cells, unless one assumes that such cells modulate rapidly in the new environment. First of all, the morphology of the alveolar macrophage is distinct from that of the Kupffer cell. Second, the aerobic metabolism and enzyme content of alveolar macrophages vary considerably from those of all other macrophages. Finally, results of the *in vitro* studies of Bennett (1966, 1967) indicate that all macrophages can be placed in three groups on the basis of various properties including cultural characteristics, and that alveolar macrophages and Kupffer cells belong to distinct physiological groups. Alveolar macrophages belong to the group characterized by a relatively high mitotic rate and the ability to attach and spread readily on glass. The second group, to which peritoneal macrophages and blood monocytes belong, attach and spread readily on glass, but have a low mitotic rate. The third group, consisting of fixed macrophages from the bone marrow, spleen, and liver, attach and spread slowly on glass but have a relatively high rate of mitosis. Thus Kupffer cells are characterized by slow attachment and spreading on glass, whereas alveolar macrophages attach and spread rapidly. Other notable dissimilarities between alveolar macrophages and Kupffer cells are differences in metabolic patterns. On the whole, the evidence does not favor the concept that appreciable numbers of Kupffer cells migrate to the lungs.

As previously mentioned, T_6 cell transfer studies in mice have indicated that, whereas two thirds of alveolar macrophages arise from transfused marrow cells, the remaining one third is derived from existing pulmonary tissue (Pinkett, Cowdrey, and Nowell, 1966). Additional evidence that substantial numbers of these cells normally arise from division of existing alveolar macrophages has been reviewed by Bertalanffy (1964).

In their studies on brain macrophages, Kosunen, Waksman, and Samuelsson (1963) found that blood-borne cells differentiate into histiocytes in the lesions of experimental allergic encephalomyelitis. By tritiated-thymidine labeling, Konigsmark and Sidman (1963) showed that circulating leukocytes were a major source of macrophages at the site of a stab wound in the brain. However, during the first 2 days of wound healing some macrophages were derived from cells already present in the brain. It seems likely that under ordinary circumstances division of preexisting brain macrophages is sufficient to account for the maintenance of normal numbers of these cells.

D. The Controversy Concerning Lymphocyte-to-Macrophage Transformation

The extensive literature pro and con on the transformation of lymphocytes into macrophages has been reviewed in great detail by Rebuck and Crowley (1955). As early as 1888, Metchnikoff noted that hematogenous lymphocytes migrate into tuberculous lesions of rodents with experimental tuberculosis. Lymphocytes in the lesions were alleged to differentiate into macrophages, epithelioid cells, and giant cells. Numerous workers have repeated these claims, as documented in the review quoted above.

Celloidin chambers implanted in tissues were employed by Maximow (1903) to study inflammation, healing, and scar formation. From the results of a series of observations, extending over the period from 5 hours to 8 months after the initiation of inflammation, Maximow concluded that macrophages are formed by transformation of blood-borne lymphocytes as well as by division of sessile histiocytes. These observations were originally challenged on the basis that lymphocytes are nonmotile and hence are unable to migrate into inflamed regions, a thesis that is no longer tenable.

Cappell (1929b) described the characteristics of cells of the omentum and mesentery, as observed by the use of vital staining. Macrophages were aggregated around vessels. Many cells resembling lymphocytes were believed to be reserves of relatively undifferentiated cells. Other cells were presumed to be intermediate between these "lymphocytes" and mature macrophages. The *taches laiteuses,* or "milk spots," are found throughout the omentum and mesentery. They are not associated with blood vessels, but are usually connected with fine lymphatic channels. Following RES stimulation, lymphocyte-like cells from the milk spots were alleged to differentiate into typical mature macrophages (Cappell, 1930). Later EM observations by Carr (1967) are in agreement with this concept.

Subsequent to the development of satisfactory cell culture techniques, Bloom (1928) reported that cells of thoracic duct lymph, predominately small lymphocytes, transform *in vitro* to monocytes, then to typical macrophages, and finally to "fibroblast-like" cells. Similar experiments using lymphocytes from other sources have been repeated by many investigators, and although some have agreed with the interpretation of Bloom (1928,

1938b), others have argued that macrophages and fibroblasts contaminate the thoracic duct lymph and that they eventually overgrow and replace dying lymphocytes. These experiments have been reviewed by Trowell (1965). Rebuck and Crowley (1955) presented data, obtained with the skin-window technique, which supports the theory that lymphocytes can transform to macrophages. They reported that during acute inflammation resting tissue histiocytes divide and give rise to an increased number of macrophages; however, the greatest share of the increase appeared to stem from intense proliferation of either blood monocytes or lymphocytes, or both.

Although the concept of lymphocyte-to-macrophage transformation is still open to question, recent reports of both *in vitro* and *in vivo* experiments lend it strong support.

Gough, Elves, and Israëls (1965) found that virtually pure preparations of blood lymphocytes did not transform into macrophages during culture *in vitro*. However, when a small proportion of neutrophils was mixed with the purified preparation of lymphocytes, much lymphocyte-to-macrophage transformation occurred. These results strongly suggest that the lymphocyte-to-macrophage transformation, presumed to occur *in vivo,* depends on homeostatic control by neutrophils or their degradation products.

Howard (1964) performed experiments *in vivo,* which strongly support the concept that lymphocytes can give rise to macrophages under certain conditions of intense RES stimulation, such as a graft-versus-host reaction. Parental thoracic duct lymphocytes with a chromosome marker were transfused into F_1 hybrids. Later, examination of Kupffer cells of the recipient showed that large numbers bore the marker and hence were derived from donor cells.

In agreement with other workers (Volkman and Gowans, 1965b), Howard, Boak, and Christie (1966) and Boak *et al.* (1968) reported that under normal conditions most macrophages in division are of bone marrow origin. However, in syngeneic radiation chimeras produced with thoracic duct cells, it was shown that during RES stimulation brought about by administration of *Corynebacterium parvum* vaccine, approximately two thirds of the liver macrophages in division were derived from chromosome-marked donor cells. Although the many nondividing cells could not be identified as to origin, the results showed decisively that thoracic duct cells, which are chiefly small lymphocytes, can give rise to macrophages during conditions of intense RES stimulation.

It would appear that the lymphocyte-to-macrophage controversy rests, at least in part, on a problem of cell heterogeneity and nomenclature. The term "small lymphocyte" is used to designate a small (6 to 8 μ) cell with a dense network of nuclear chromatin, surrounded by a thin rim of cytoplasm. These cells are normally found in blood, lymph, and lymphoid tissues. However, the morphological definition, small lymphocyte, has no implications with respect to heritage or ultimate fate, but simply designates an inactive resting cell with most of its genome repressed. It seems probable that small lymphocytes merely represent resting cells of heterogeneous origins and potentialities (Berman, 1966; Volkman, 1966) and that they can respond to different stimuli by differentiating to various cell types. Although there is good evidence that some of these cells recirculate for months or years (Everett and Tyler, 1967) it is known that some can respond to certain stimuli with derepression and differentiation (Gowans and McGregor, 1965). For example, many, but not all, lymphocytes respond to phytohemagglutinin (PHA) with blast transformation. Their nuclei become activated and histones are acetylated (Pogo, Allfrey, and Mirsky, 1966). Nucleoli form, which probably serve as the site of ribosomal synthesis, and greatly increased numbers of ribosomes cause increased basophilia of the cytoplasm. Such blast cells can in turn divide and give rise to small lymphocytes.

Elves (1967) presented data which suggest that at least two populations of lymphocytes exist: one which can be stimulated to undergo blast transformation, and another which has the capacity to differentiate into macrophages in the presence of PMNs. As previously stated, it is presumed that the transformation of lymphocytes to macrophages is initiated by products of dying PMNs. This could readily explain the sequence of cellular changes in inflammatory exudates.

The existence of more than one population of lymphocytes was also suggested by the data of Berman and Stulberg (1962), who reported that human buffy coat cultures after 15 to 25 days *in vitro* consist almost entirely of macrophages, giant cells, and small lymphocytes. Presumably many of the macrophages in the cultures arose from small lymphocytes. When PHA was added to the 15- to 25-day-old cultures, the remaining lymphocytes underwent blastogenesis. These results indicate that in the presence of PMNs some of the lymphocytes in blood are capable of transforming into macrophages, and that other lymphocytes lack this capacity but are able to respond to PHA with blast transformation.

Even if some small lymphocytes have the capacity to differentiate into macrophages following appropriate stimuli, there is no reason to believe that all lymphocytes have this capacity. Since macrophages evidently do not form antibodies, it is also reasonable to suppose that any lymphocyte progenitor of macrophages would likewise be incapable of forming antibodies. Better techniques for cell identification ultimately may permit more precise classification of small lymphocytes than is possible with morphological criteria alone. For example, if a population of cells exists with the morphology of lymphocytes and the potential of differentiating

into macrophages, its members may already possess certain characteristics of macrophages such as cytophilic antibody receptors on their surfaces. This would permit the distinction of these cells from lymphocytes
with other potentialities, such as hematopoietic capabilities or the capacity
to respond to antigens with blast transformation.

To recapitulate, the controversy about a possible lymphocyte-to-macrophage transformation remains open. The strength of evidence indicates
that some, but certainly not all, cells with the morphology of small
lymphocytes can respond *in vitro* to the presence of PMNs by transforming into macrophages. The *in vivo* circumstances in which such a transformation is claimed to occur invariably involve the presence of PMNs
(see Chapter 5).

SUMMARY: Evidence is cited in support of the bone marrow origin
of most of the macrophages normally found in lung, peritoneal exudate,
and local inflammatory lesions. There is general agreement that monocytes migrate from the circulation and mature into typical tissue and
exudative macrophages. Other potential sources of macrophages include
mobilization and proliferation of existing tissue macrophages, migration
of Kupffer cells into the lung, the transformation of lymphocytes to
macrophages, and the remote possibility that macrophages may arise
by differentiation of specialized endothelium. The controversy concerning lymphocyte-to-macrophage transformation is discussed. Most of the
available data are consistent with the concept that some lymphocytes can
transform into macrophages under the homeostatic control of PMNs or
their degradation products.

Chapter 5

Macrophages and Cellular Homeostasis

THE PROBLEM of determining the factors responsible for cell differentiation and homeostasis in complex organisms is currently one of the most fascinating aspects of biological research. Macrophages function in the homeostasis of several cell types in higher animals, while other cells influence macrophage proliferation and differentiation.

A. General Theories Concerning Homeostasis

Recently several interesting hypotheses relating to the overall problem of homeostasis have been set forth. Burwell (1963) and Burch and Burwell (1965) postulated that "tissue coding factors" (TCF) released from tissues reach regional lymph nodes where they may be processed by macrophages before being presented to lymphoid cells. They proposed that, by reacting with specific cell-bound receptor molecules on the surfaces of mitotically competent lymphoid cells, TCF enables these cells to regulate tissue growth throughout the mammalian organism. According to another theory, formulated by Heinmets (1968), exoenzymes on cell membranes of macrophages or other cells act on substrates on the surfaces of adjacent cells. It is proposed that the products of substrate degradation are carried into the exoenzyme-bearing cells where they can act as operon activators to control synthetic processes. Strong experimental evidence to support these hypotheses has not been presented.

One of the best examples of the *modus operandi* of cell differentiation and homeostasis in adult mammals is the development of erythropoietic and lymphoid tissue. The existence of undifferentiated stem cells as progenitors of certain cell types is well known, although their morphology has not been established. A bone marrow cell morphologically similar to the lymphocyte may serve as the stem cell for erythroid and lymphoid tissue (Yoffey *et al.,* 1961). It is probable that the bone marrow stem cell is multipotent (Trentin and co-workers, 1967). Virolainen and Defendi (1968) presented findings which suggest that a single bone marrow stem cell can give rise to cells of the erythrocytic, lymphocytic, and monocytic series. Alternatively, more than one bone marrow stem cell population may exist (Boggs, 1966). There is also evidence to support the concept that the lymphocytic series is distinct from the plasmacytic series, as suggested by Fagraeus (1948). For example, patients with hereditary sex-linked agammaglobulinemia are deficient in cells of the plasmacytic, but not the lymphocytic, series. Additional evidence indicating that the two series of cells are distinct has been presented by Storb and Weiser (1968), as the result of studies on the cellular kinetics of antibody production.

There is general agreement that the stem cell progenitors of erythroid and lymphoid cells, as well as macrophages, are located chiefly in the bone marrow, although they may also be found in lymph nodes (Ford, Micklem, and Ogden, 1968). The possibility that a common stem cell serves as the progenitor of both lymphocytic elements and macrophages is still open to question.

Factors which control the proliferation and differentiation of stem cells are under intensive investigation. Bullough (1965, 1967) has discussed much of the pertinent literature. The differentiation of bone marrow stem cells into erythrocytes under the influence of erythropoietin is a good model of cell differentiation. The hormone erythropoietin is formed in the kidney during conditions which cause anoxia, and results in an outpouring of erythrocytes into the peripheral circulation. Similar inducers for the production of granulocytes and macrophages have been postulated, but not demonstrated. The model of homeostasis in erythrocyte production has permitted a study of feedback regulation. Polycythemia produced passively with syngeneic, allogeneic, or even xenogeneic erythrocytes inhibits the ability of bone marrow cells transplanted into lethally x-irradiated recipients to supply progenitors of erythroid clones (Feldman and Bleiberg, 1967). In sublethally irradiated animals as well, polycythemia inhibits the formation of erythroid clones from endogenous cells, owing to suppression of the production of erythropoietin. As expected, this condition can be reversed by the administration of erythropoietin, which acts on the progeny of the transfused stem cells. In the absence of erythropoietin, stem cells can replicate but erythroid colonies are not formed. Other evidence indicating that stem cells must differentiate to a point where they are committed to erythropoiesis before the hormone can act on them has come from the work of O'Grady, Lewis, and Trobaugh (1968), who showed that erythropoietin is required for the maturation of erythroid tissue, but not for differentiation of stem cells.

The extent to which de-differentiation of the cells of higher animals may serve to provide precursor cells is not known. It has generally been assumed that genome repression in differentiated cells of vertebrates is irreversible; however, such repression in highly differentiated cells can be abated under certain experimental conditions. Gurdon and Uehlinger (1966) transplanted nuclei from differentiated intestinal cells of *Xenopus* feeding tadpoles into enucleated *Xenopus* ova and showed that fully mature fertile male and female frogs developed from such ova. This indicates that the state of genome repression, in higher animals as well as in simple organisms, depends on environmental conditions both within and outside the cell. Thus, differentiation can be reversed under appropriate circumstances. A major unsolved problem is that of determining the nature of the specific inducers and repressors involved in differentiation and de-differentiation. For example, if a stem cell can give rise to either a lymphocyte, a plasma cell, or a macrophage, what are the environmental stimuli that account for the differentiation to one or the other of these cell types?

Clear evidence of genome derepression in differentiated cells has been provided by Harris (1966), who showed that the cytoplasm is responsible for the functional state of the nucleus it encloses. Harris used Sendai virus to fuse cell membranes of human or mouse fibroblasts with membranes of avian erythrocyte ghosts containing a nucleus but essentially no cytoplasm. The heterokaryon made, for example, from a HeLa cell fused with an avian erythrocyte ghost, consists of a large human HeLa cell nucleus and a small erythrocyte nucleus, both surrounded by HeLa cell cytoplasm. Within this environment the normally inactive red cell nucleus soon begins to enlarge, the condensed chromatin becomes disperse, and ribonucleic acid (RNA) synthesis begins. After a time, nucleoli form and avian proteins are synthesized. These experiments clearly showed that human cytoplasmic elements can activate the avian nucleus, and that the environment within the cell determines the state of activity of the nucleus. It is important to stress that gene expression probably depends even more upon the environment within the cell than upon the extracellular milieu (Markert, 1963).

Mouse spleen or bone marrow cells can proliferate *in vitro* to form colonies in agar (Pluznik and Sachs, 1966; Bradley and Metcalf, 1966). The influence of the extracellular environment on cell proliferation and differentiation within clones of bone marrow cells was demonstrated by the work of Metcalf, Bradley, and Robinson (1967). In these experiments, when mouse bone marrow cells were stimulated by either kidney feeder layers or leukemic serum the colonies which developed were at first granulocytic but later became predominately monocytic. It was suggested that the granulocytic colonies arose from the proliferation of single cells, and that adjacent primitive mononuclear cells trapped in the agar were influenced by contact with the growing colonies. It was postulated that the microenvironment of the granulocytic colonies stimulated proliferation of progenitors of mononuclear cells, which then formed colonies of phagocytic mononuclear cells.

A growth regulator of singular interest has been described by Bullough and Laurence (1967) and Bullough *et al.* (1967), who extracted an anti-mitotic substance from the epidermis of the mouse, man, and even codfish which acts on epidermal cells of the same and other species. This substance, called epidermal chalone, is tissue-specific but acts across wide species barriers, and appears to be a low molecular weight glycoprotein with basic properties. Tissue-specific chalones have been extracted from liver, kidney, and granulocytes, and it is reasonable to assume that similar mitosis-regulating substances exist for other cell types, including the macrophage.

It has been postulated by Bullough that during the healing of skin wounds the concentration of mitosis-inhibiting chalone within epidermal cells is reduced owing to fluid uptake by the cells, with a consequent increase in epidermal mitosis. Following replacement of destroyed epidermal cells, mitosis would cease because the level of chalones again becomes normal. It is assumed that the lower the chalone concentration, the more active is the mitosis operon and the more rapid the onset of synthesis of enzymes essential to mitosis.

These general theories of homeostasis have not been tested experimentally in the macrophage system; however, certain lipids and hormones appear to play important roles in macrophage homeostasis. There is also evidence to suggest that interactions between macrophages and other cells play an important part in maintaining homeostasis of the interacting cells.

B. *Factors Influencing Macrophage Proliferation and Differentiation*

Substances which are known to influence macrophage differentiation and proliferation are discussed below.

1. Lipids

The abundant evidence that lipids affect the phagocytic capacity of macrophages will be discussed elsewhere. Certain lipids also influence macrophage proliferation. Stanley (1949; 1950) extracted a chloroform-soluble lipid called monocytosis-producing agent (MPA) from *Listeria monocytogenes,* an organism so named because of the characteristic mono-cytosis that it produces in mammalian hosts. Stanley showed that MPA can produce monocytosis in animals. Lipids from tubercle bacilli and other mycobacteria also elicit monocytosis and granulomatous responses (reviewed by Canetti, 1955). The chemical nature of these monocyto-genic lipids has not been determined.

2. Endotoxins

Endotoxins exert an influence on macrophages, but the manner in which this influence is mediated is uncertain. The results of endotoxin treatment are so extremely diverse that it is difficult to determine the mechanisms of action leading to any one effect (see Chapter 7, Section F).

Windle *et al.* (1950) studied the effects of a *Pseudomonas* endotoxin on the cells and tissues of a variety of laboratory animals. They reported that the most consistent alteration observed following endotoxin treatment was hyperplasia and sometimes metaplasia of the lymphoid and myeloid organs. Small repeated doses of endotoxin given over a short period of time led to increased phagocytosis. More intensive treatment over longer periods of time resulted in the accumulation of large numbers of macrophages and lymphocytes in spleen, lymph nodes, and bone marrow. Thus, although the mechanism of action is unknown, it would appear that endotoxin administration can lead to extensive proliferation of various types of cells, including macrophages.

A later report of Windle *et al.* (1954) may also be significant. Although spinal cord transection is almost universally irreparable there has been a report of limited restoration of function in a patient infected with gram-negative bacilli. It was postulated that endotoxin from gram-negative organisms might inhibit scarring and permit nerve regeneration in the cord. To test this hypothesis, Windle and co-workers subjected adult cats with upper lumbar cord transection to endotoxin treatment. They reported a temporary limited restoration of nerve function in some of the animals. Eventually, the formation of scars led to loss of function of the regenerated cord. These results suggest that macrophages and fibroblasts exert a homeostatic influence on each other and that, when macrophage function is impaired, fibroblast proliferation, healing, and scarring are inhibited. However, it is also possible that some other effect of endotoxin may have led to these interesting results.

In general, endotoxins play an ill-defined role in macrophage homeostasis. They destroy macrophages under certain conditions, but can also lead to macrophage proliferation; dosage and timing of endotoxin administration are of primary importance. Through their action on macrophages, endotoxins could affect homeostasis of other cell types as well. Whether indirect effects of endotoxin, such as hormone alterations, contribute to their overall activity to any extent is not known.

3. Monocytogenic Hormone

Willoughby, Coote, and Spector (1967) reported that the injection of Freund's complete adjuvant directly into lymph nodes is followed by a marked and prolonged monocytosis (three to ten times the normal number of circulating monocytes) lasting for 6 weeks or longer. They postulated that a monocytogenic hormone, produced by the stimulated lymphoid tissue, probably acts on bone marrow, since the active factor could be transferred with serum. These authors suggested that this monocytogenic hormone causes proliferation of macrophages during states of delayed sensitivity.

4. Other Agents

Substances which are lethal for macrophages have the final result of causing their compensatory proliferation. For example, crystalline silica (see Section C) and the radioactive compound thorium dioxide (Thorotrast) are both extremely toxic for macrophages (Mims, 1964b). When administered in large doses they cause death of macrophages, followed by a compensatory macrophage proliferation.

During macrophage proliferation, changes occur which appear to involve more than a simple derepression of the genome leading to mitosis. It is known that increased demand for macrophages, however it may be signaled, has several results. First, macrophages are mobilized from depots near the site where they are needed. Second, immature monocytes infiltrate the site and mature into tissue or exudative macrophages. Third, bone marrow or other stem cells are stimulated, perhaps by hormone action, to proliferate and differentiate into monocytes, which enter the circulation and finally sequestrate and mature into macrophages. Each of these events is probably controlled by some independent stimulus or by the interaction of several stimuli. The problem offers a challenging field for further investigation.

C. Cellular Interrelationships

1. Macrophage and Plasma Cell

As mentioned above, crystalline silica is highly toxic for macrophages. *In vivo* studies in many animal species have shown that a marked granulomatous response follows the initial destruction of macrophages by silica (Vigliani and Pernis, 1961; 1963). An adjuvant effect on humoral antibody production has also been reported in silica-treated animals exposed to antigens (Ghiringhelli and Pernis, 1958; Antweiler, 1959). A conspicuous proliferation of lymphoid and plasma cells is observed in the popliteal lymph nodes following the injection of a lysate of rabbit macrophages into the footpads of rabbits (Mollo and Governa, 1961). A similar plasmacytic proliferation is observed in silicotic nodules where macrophage destruction has occurred. In instances in which foreign antigens are included in the injected material the plasmacytic stimulation could account for the increased serum and tissue levels of specific antibodies. In instances in which only silica or macrophage lysates are injected the plasmacytic response could be due to foreign antigens which may fortuitously be present in macrophages, perhaps processed as "super-antigens" (see Chapter 9). Although the mechanisms concerned in the interaction between macrophages and cells of the plasmacytic series are unknown, macrophages appear to exert a homeostatic effect on plasma cells, at least under certain conditions.

2. Lymphocyte and Macrophage

Transfused cells of thoracic duct lymph, virtually all of which have the morphology of lymphocytes, can repopulate the liver and other tissues with macrophages during periods of intense RES stimulation (Boak *et al.,* 1968). The possible role of lymphocytes as regular precursors of macrophages, or as cells capable of differentiating or transforming into mature macrophages, has been discussed in some detail in Chapter 4, Section D.

Aside from a possible precursor role, lymphocytes do not appear to influence macrophage proliferation to a significant extent. For example, following sublethal x-irradiation, lymphocytes are depleted in blood and tissues; however, there is no evidence that macrophage homeostasis is substantially affected. Gallily and Feldman (1966; 1967a, b) and Feldman and Gallily (1967) reported that antigen processing by macrophages may be adversely affected by x-irradiation; however, phagocytic capabilities and homeostasis of macrophages did not appear to be disturbed.

3. Macrophage and Fibroblast

Enlightenment on the relationship of macrophages with other cell types has been provided by studies of pathological conditions such as silicosis. For centuries it has been known that a relationship exists between dust exposure and lung disease (Agricola, 1556), and that pulmonary fibrosis occurs as the result of exposure to a wide variety of dusts. With increased mining of coal and minerals during the past century, pulmonary fibrosis became a major public health problem. Attempts to solve this problem resulted in studies on the pneumoconioses which have led to the following concepts of the relationship between macrophages and fibroblasts.

Crystalline silicon dioxide (silica) is present in most fibrogenic dusts. This substance, SiO_2, occurs in amorphous as well as crystalline forms; however, only the latter are fibrogenic. Two of the forms of crystalline silica are quartz, which makes up almost 60% of the earth's crust, and tridymite, which is rare in nature but is even more fibrogenic than quartz (King *et al.,* 1953). Studies of tissue sections from patients with silicosis and from laboratory animals exposed to silica-containing dusts revealed that extensive necrosis of macrophages occurs subsequent to phagocytosis of the dust particles. This macrophage necrosis is followed by a characteristic cellular reaction and ultimate fibrosis (Vigliani and Pernis, 1961; Harington, 1963).

Although silica is phagocytized by a number of cell types, including PMNs, it is selectively toxic for macrophages (Kessel, Monaco, and Marchisio, 1963). The toxicity depends not only on crystalline form, but also on particle size, particles 0.5 μ and smaller being the most toxic (Hatch and Kindsvatter, 1947). Contact between silica particles and macrophage is required for toxicity; silica enclosed in diffusion chambers

in vivo is innocuous (Curran and Rowsell, 1958). The relation of crystalline form to cytotoxicity of silica particles is of interest. Recent *in vitro*
experiments using electron microscopy and enzyme histochemical pro-
cedures have disclosed the probable mechanism of macrophage destruction
by silica (Allison, Harington, and Birbeck, 1966; Comolli, 1967). Evidently phagocytized silica particles act on phagolysosomal membranes and
allow leakage of hydrolytic enzymes into the cytoplasm, and eventually
into the medium, resulting in cell death. The selectivity of crystalline silica
for macrophage membranes suggests that the crystals may interact with
some specific chemical configuration peculiar to macrophage membranes.
Upon lysis of the cell, the silica is liberated and is soon phagocytized by
other macrophages. Cycling of the silica, which cannot be metabolized,
results in a prolonged period of macrophage destruction. After a time,
usually months or years, the cycle ends when fibrosis finally walls off the
offending particles in granulomatous lesions.

Fibroblasts are present in silicotic lesions from their inception and
rapidly increase in numbers. Collagen production is marked and as much
as 40% of the total protein of the silicotic nodule is collagen (Pernis, 1955).
The necrosis of macrophages which could be observed in tissue sections
prior to fibroblast proliferation strongly suggested that some factor released from dying mature macrophages induces fibroblast proliferation
and collagen synthesis. Confirmation of this concept has come from experiments *in vitro* which have shown that a factor released from dying rat
peritoneal macrophages after silica ingestion causes increased fibrogenesis
by chick embryo fibroblasts (Heppleston and Styles, 1967).

With respect to the role of the macrophage in the homeostasis of fibroblasts, it is of interest that there have been reports of reticulum cell sarcomas apparently caused by long-term RES stimulation. Gillman, Gillman,
and Gilbert (1949) noted that reticulum cell sarcomas develop in the livers
of rats following prolonged treatment with trypan blue. The work of Simpson (1952) confirmed this observation. Gillman and co-workers (1949)
found that cysts and tumors were frequently formed in the liver, apparently
by rapidly proliferating malignant histiocytes, and once formed they remained for many months. The absence of fibrosis was very remarkable in
such livers. A probable explanation to account for this phenomenon is that
immature neoplastic macrophages lack the capacity to synthesize the
inducer of fibrosis.

A macrophage growth factor (MGF) produced by fibroblasts has been
characterized by Virolainen and Defendi (1967), who found that culture
medium removed from 3-day cultures of L-cells or mouse embryo fibroblasts serves to stimulate the proliferation of mouse macrophages *in vitro*.
Medium collected from syngeneic or allogeneic, but not xenogeneic, fibroblasts was effective. It was possible to maintain macrophage cultures for

several cell divisions, provided MGF was added regularly. The factor was stable at 65° C for 1 hour but lost activity when heated to 100° C for 10 minutes. Activity was fully maintained during storage for 6 months at 4° C, but when held at 37° C for 6 months there was some loss of activity. It was not dialyzable, either before or after trypsin treatment, and it was resistant to a wide variety of hydrolytic enzymes. Activity was not destroyed by treatment with ether or with ultraviolet light for 30 minutes. It is possible that MGF is identical or closely related to the macrophage inducer described by Ichikawa, Pluznik, and Sachs (1966, 1967) and discussed below.

4. Polymorphonuclear Neutrophil and Macrophage

Homeostasis of normal mouse macrophages and granulocytes has been studied in an *in vitro* system by Pluznik and Sachs (1966) and Ichikawa, Pluznik, and Sachs (1966, 1967). It was found that cultured fibroblasts and some other types of cells release a substance(s) which can induce the formation of colonies of macrophages or granulocytes from single cells of embryo liver or adult spleen. The inducer substance was nondialyzable and stable at 37° C for at least a week. It lost only 30% of its activity after heating at 56° C for 30 minutes, but lost all activity after heating at 90° C for 30 minutes. Subsequent experiments revealed that the ability of the substance to induce macrophage colony formation from progenitor cells is inhibited in the presence of irradiated macrophage feeder layers. This was shown to be due to a dialyzable inhibitor substance produced by the macrophages (Ichikawa *et al.,* 1967). Although the inducer substance was required for formation of colonies of either macrophages or granulocytes, the inhibitor substance formed by irradiated macrophages inhibited macrophage colony growth only. It was proposed that the system represents a mechanism for homeostatic control of growth and development of macrophages and granulocytes; the inducer for both types of cells being produced by fibroblasts, and the inhibitor for macrophages being produced by mature macrophages.

There is evidence that granulocytes contain a factor(s) which causes cells resembling small lymphocytes to transform into macrophages. Gough, Elves, and Israëls (1965) found that blood lymphocytes alone did not transform into macrophages *in vitro;* however, if granulocytes were added to purified lymphocytes, extensive transformation occurred.

Other evidence in support of PMN stimulation of macrophage differentiation has come from the work of Jones (1966). When mixed cultures of genetically dissimilar blood leukocytes are prepared, many macrophages are present at 3 days and many blast cells are seen at 6 to 9 days. On the other hand, when most of the PMNs are removed from the blood before mixed cultures are prepared, they contain relatively small numbers of macrophages at 3 days and blast cells at 6 to 9 days. It was suggested that PMNs induce some lymphocytes to transform to macrophages which can then take up foreign leukocyte antigens and present them to lymphocytes, resulting in an increase in blast transformation. Apparently monocytes, PMNs, and lymphocytes exert a mutual regulatory influence on their differentiation and activities. Such an interaction could contribute substantially to the cellular changes observed during an inflammatory response.

5. Macrophage and Macrophage

Interaction of normal cells leads to contact inhibition *in vitro*. This is true of macrophages, as well as other cell types. Whether this phenomenon has any relevance to homeostasis *in vivo* is not known, although it would be expected.

As discussed in Section 4 above, macrophages have been shown to produce an inhibitor which counteracts macrophage-inducer substances. Thus macrophage-macrophage interaction would appear to be of major importance in homeostasis of this cell type.

SUMMARY: The general subject of homeostasis is discussed briefly, and several hypotheses and model systems are mentioned, especially in relation to homeostasis concerning macrophages. Certain substances known to influence macrophage proliferation and differentiation include lipids, endotoxins, a monocytogenic hormone, silicon dioxide, and thorium dioxide. Cellular interactions also profoundly affect homeostasis. The interrelationships between various cell types, both *in vitro* and *in vivo,* are discussed. It is apparent that mutual regulatory influences between granulocytes, lymphocytes, macrophages, plasma cells, and fibroblasts could profoundly affect the cellular changes observed during the inflammatory response.

Chapter 6

Macrophage Metabolism

MANY MACROPHAGES have a high degree of metabolic activity. Largely by the use of *in vitro* techniques, it has been shown that peritoneal and alveolar macrophages differ in their metabolic patterns and enzyme loads and that certain macrophages perform specialized metabolic activities.

A. Metabolic Requirements in Vitro

Macrophages can be maintained for short periods *in vitro* without difficulty. They retain many of their morphological characteristics and properties, such as phagocytic ability, while in culture (cf. review by Jacoby, 1965). Under special conditions they can be cultured over long periods of time; Chang (1964) reported that mouse peritoneal macrophages can be maintained *in vitro* for as long as 220 days.

Macrophages ingest nutrients from the medium either by phagocytosis or pinocytosis. For example, dilute serum is actively ingested by monolayers of chick macrophages over a period of several hours; consequently the cells become highly vacuolated during the first day in culture. The pinocytized material is digested by the cells, and extensive pinocytosis does not occur again until fresh medium is added (Jacoby, 1965).

Macrophages can be maintained in relatively simple culture media, such as complete Hanks' medium or Medium 199, if serum is added. The concentration of serum used for successful short-term maintenance of macrophages can be varied considerably. Although 10 to 25% serum is customarily used, as much as 50 to 100% of the medium can be serum (Rous and Beard, 1934; Beard and Rous, 1934; Cohn and Parks, 1967 a,b,c). Calf serum is usually satisfactory for the cultivation of rat and mouse macrophages, but sera of other species may be toxic. Jacoby (1965) summarized much of the literature on serum requirements of macrophages and the toxicity of xenogeneic sera.

Cohn and Benson (1965c) noted that protein synthesis by mouse peritoneal macrophages was greatly increased when the amount of fetal calf serum in the medium was increased from 1 to 20%. Similarly, Stecher and Thorbecke (1967b) found that both rat and mouse peritoneal macrophages synthesize much more β_{1C} globulin and transferrin when the medium contains 20% newborn calf serum rather than 1% serum. Macrophages of the rat, but not the mouse, were able to synthesize certain serum proteins in a synthetic medium containing 0.1 to 0.2 μg/ml of hydrocortisone in lieu of serum; higher concentrations (1 μg/ml) of hydrocortisone completely inhibited synthesis. It was postulated that cortisol, which is naturally bound to albumin in the serum, is slowly released and acts as a membrane stabilizer or in some other way to profoundly affect metabolism.

Macrophages have not been grown in completely synthetic media without cortisone. Even when the medium contains serum, macrophages may have limited metabolic potential. As a rule, macrophage proliferation is sparse or absent in ordinary culture media (Jacoby, 1965; Bennett, 1966); however, it can be induced in several ways. One procedure is to add macrophage growth factor to the culture. This factor, described by Virolainen and Defendi (1967), is present in medium collected from cultures of syngeneic or allogeneic (but not xenogeneic) fibroblasts. Proliferation can also be induced with appropriate amounts of endotoxin (Forbes, 1965), or by means of an antigen-antibody reaction (Forbes and Mackaness, 1963; Rowley and Leuchtenberger, 1964; Forbes, 1966). Macrophages from sensitized animals can respond *in vitro* to specific antigen with mitosis and proliferation, evidently by virtue of cytophilic antibodies which combine with the antigen at the cell surface.

B. Energy Sources

1. Peritoneal Macrophages

The *in vitro* studies of Harris and Barclay (1955) showed that rabbit peritoneal macrophages are facultative anaerobes. In the presence of oxygen, they had a constant O_2 uptake which did not depend on the oxygen tension of the medium. Most of the glucose used was converted to lactic acid, even when O_2 was present. Increased glycolysis supplied cellular energy requirements under anaerobic conditions. The conclusion drawn was that the metabolism of peritoneal macrophages depends largely on energy obtained by glycolysis under either aerobic or anaerobic conditions. Similar conclusions were reached by Oren *et al.* (1963), who found that peritoneal macrophages of the guinea pig depend on glycolysis as the principal source of energy for phagocytosis.

Energy for pinocytosis may be derived in other ways. Cohn (1966) demonstrated that the high degree of pinocytosis exhibited by mouse peritoneal macrophages cultured in 50% newborn calf serum can be markedly reduced by a number of metabolic inhibitors. The most effective inhibition of pinocytosis was achieved with cyanide, antimycin A, or anaerobiosis, thus indicating that these cells depend largely on mitochondrial activity for energy to support extensive pinocytosis.

Thus, peritoneal macrophages are facultative anaerobes which utilize glycolysis as a major metabolic pathway. They are also capable of obtaining energy via aerobic metabolism in certain circumstances.

2. Alveolar Macrophages

It is generally agreed that alveolar macrophages are facultative aerobes. Oren et al. (1963) compared the metabolism of alveolar macrophages, peritoneal macrophages, and peritoneal PMNs of the guinea pig. They showed that resting alveolar macrophages have a much higher level of oxygen uptake than does either of the other two cell types. Furthermore, inhibitors of oxidative phosphorylation suppressed phagocytosis by alveolar macrophages, indicating that these cells depend on aerobic oxidative metabolism for the energy used in phagocytosis (see Chapter 7, Section C).

The metabolism of alveolar macrophages of rabbits has been investigated by Ouchi, Selvaraj, and Sbarra (1965). In agreement with the work just discussed, the results of these investigators indicated that noninduced alveolar macrophages utilize aerobic metabolism to supply the energy required for phagocytosis. Inhibitors of the tricarboxylic acid (TCA) cycle did not inhibit phagocytosis, even though it was shown that they enter the cells, indicating that the TCA cycle is not a major source of energy for phagocytosis by these alveolar macrophages. It was subsequently shown by Myrvik and Evans (1967a, b) that, following challenge of sensitized rabbits with BCG, there is a large increase in hexose monophosphate shunt metabolism by macrophages.

Thus it would appear that the energy requirements of alveolar macrophages are normally met by oxidative metabolism. The production of energy required for phagocytosis will be further discussed in Chapter 7.

C. Synthesis of Enzymes

From the time of Metchnikoff it has been recognized that macrophages contain cytoplasmic granules which stain with neutral red, and that activated macrophages contain more of these granules than do nonactivated macrophages. Cappell (1929a, b, c) studied the principles and techniques of neutral red staining. He noted that neutral red is basic and stains the granules of macrophages in a characteristic manner. By use of the more sophisticated techniques of histochemistry and electron microscopy, North (1966b) showed that acid phosphatase is abundant in the lysosomes of macrophages and that, following fusion of phagosomes with lysosomes, the enzyme is discharged into phagolysosomes. That the enzymes in macrophage lysosomes are actively synthesized by the cell is apparent from the studies of Cohn and Benson (1965b), in which metabolic inhibitors and radioactive labels were used.

Macrophages not only contain large quantities of acid hydrolases enclosed within lysosomes, but also show characteristic patterns of enzyme activity (see review by Cohn, 1965). Indeed, Braunstein, Freiman, and

Gall (1958) suggested that the characteristic pattern of enzyme activity might prove to be as reliable an indicator for distinguishing macrophages from other cells in certain mixed cell populations as the silver stain described by Marshall (1956).

The enzyme loads of macrophages can vary considerably, depending on the regional source of the cells, the stimulus to their proliferation or maturation, and other factors. Because the cell populations studied frequently have been from either peritoneum, lung, blood, or other tissues, it is possible to discuss some of the evidence illustrating the enzyme pattern of each of these regional populations of macrophages.

1. Peritoneal Macrophages

Hydrolytic enzymes of the peritoneal macrophages of rabbits were assayed by Dannenberg and Bennett (1964). Lysosomes were ruptured by freezing and thawing the cells, and two proteases were characterized in the resulting lysate. The first, with a pH optimum of 4.0, is similar to the pepsin-like proteinase I of the lung; the second, with a pH optimum between 5.0 and 5.8, resembles chymotrypsin. Esterases that hydrolyze methyl butyrate and β-naphthyl acetate at pH 7.0 to 8.0 were present, as well as a lipase with a pH optimum of 6.1, which has many of the characteristics of a lipoprotein lipase previously described. Rabbit peritoneal macrophages have also been shown to contain cholesterol esterase (Day, 1960a; Day and Gould-Hurst, 1963).

Histochemical studies (Kessel et al., 1963) indicate that the macrophages of several species contain the following enzymes: succinic dehydrogenase, alkaline and acid phosphatases, esterases, aminopeptidase, lipase, DPN and TPN diaphorase, and β-glucuronidase.

Sonically disrupted peritoneal macrophages from normal rats and guinea pigs and from BCG-immunized guinea pigs were analyzed for enzyme content by Colwell, Hess, and Tavaststjerna (1963). The following enzyme activities were found: alkaline phosphatase in rat but not in guinea pig peritoneal macrophages; acid phosphatase in guinea pig and rat peritoneal macrophages; β-glucuronidase in both; lysozyme in both, but more in peritoneal macrophages from rats; esterase (tributyrinase) in peritoneal macrophages from guinea pigs but not rats; and lipase in both.

The lysozyme content of peritoneal macrophages from normal outbred rabbits is much lower than that of their alveolar macrophages (Myrvik, Leake, and Fariss, 1961b). Macrophages from normal rabbits of strains inbred for either resistance or susceptibility to tuberculosis show no substantial difference in lysozyme content; however the alveolar macrophages of normal rabbits contain about seven times as much lysozyme as their peritoneal macrophages (Carson and Dannenberg, 1965).

Following infection, the enzyme content of macrophages increases.

Carson and Dannenberg (1965) reported lysozyme levels 1.4 times normal in peritoneal macrophages collected from tuberculous rabbits. Saito and Suter (1965) found significant increases in acid phosphatase, β-glucuronidase, and cathepsin, in peritoneal macrophages from mice infected with BCG. Similar results were obtained by Heise, Myrvik, and Leake (1965) with alveolar macrophages of the rabbit.

Bennett (1966) compared the *in vitro* growth characteristics of relatively purified populations of mouse macrophages from the peritoneum, lung, and other sites. He found that the lysosomal acid phosphatase activity of peritoneal macrophages increases after 24 hours *in vitro*. Cohn and Benson (1965c) evaluated the effects of varied cultural conditions on hydrolase activity of mouse peritoneal macrophages. Little or no increase in enzyme levels occurred when small amounts of newborn calf serum were added to the culture medium; when the concentration of serum in the medium was increased, acid phosphatase, cathepsin, and β-glucuronidase were formed more rapidly and in larger amounts. Evidently, increased enzyme production was related to improved cellular function which resulted from the increased pinocytosis induced by high levels of serum.

North (1966a) demonstrated a nucleoside phosphatase, apparently ATPase, on the membrane of guinea pig peritoneal macrophages. It was postulated that the activity of this enzyme supplies energy for phagocytosis and membrane movement.

Many other enzymes have been demonstrated in the peritoneal macrophages of various species; some of these are listed in the table presented on pages 48 and 49 of this chapter.

2. Alveolar Macrophages

By virtue of their location within alveoli, lung macrophages are of prime importance in protecting the respiratory tract against microbial invasion. They are extremely rich in enzymes, some of which are known to be involved in intracellular destruction of bacteria. Myrvik, Leake, and Fariss (1961a) described a method for obtaining large quantities of relatively pure suspensions of alveolar macrophages, which has been very useful for *in vitro* studies. With this technique, approximately 0.1 to 0.2 ml of packed alveolar macrophages can be washed from the lungs of a normal rabbit. Following vaccination and subsequent challenge with tubercle bacilli the yield is tremendously increased to 2.5 to 8.0 ml packed cells (Myrvik, Leake, and Oshima, 1962).

Myrvik, Leake, and Fariss (1961b) measured lysozyme in extracts of alveolar macrophages obtained by freezing and thawing the cells. The lysozyme level in alveolar macrophages was 3400 μg/ml of packed cells; in contrast, 540 μg of lysozyme were present in each milliliter of packed peritoneal cells having a similar protein content. The authors postulated that this high content of lysozyme in alveolar macrophages from normal rabbits may be related to the capacity of the cells to destroy some of the microorganisms which commonly invade the lower respiratory tract.

Lysozyme levels in extracts of alveolar macrophages from rabbits vaccinated and challenged with tubercle bacilli of the BCG strain were five to six times normal. Furthermore, the lysozyme content of macrophage extracts paralleled their bacteriostatic activity against mycobacterial cultures (Oshima, Myrvik, and Leake, 1961). In this experimental approximation of early reinfection tuberculosis, the immunized animals react to the bacilli used for challenge with tremendous proliferation of immune alveolar macrophages. It is probable that lysozyme synthesized by such macrophages plays a major role in the immune response to the infection.

Leake and Myrvik (1964) showed that in normal rabbit alveolar macrophages the enzyme, acid phosphatase, is contained in osmotically sensitive granules possessing the general properties of classical lysosomes. The granules carrying lysozyme (probably lysosomes) were uniquely resistant to osmotic shock in distilled water and released the enzyme only when electrolyte was added.

Histochemical techniques were used by Dannenberg, Burstone, Walter, and Kinsley (1963) to assay the following six enzymes in alveolar macrophages and in peritoneal exudate cells: cytochrome oxidase, aminopeptidase, succinic dehydrogenase, acid phosphatase, alkaline phosphatase, and esterase. Alkaline phosphatase was found in neutrophils but not in alveolar or peritoneal macrophages. The other five enzymes were more abundant in alveolar than in peritoneal macrophages. Alveolar and peritoneal macrophages containing recently ingested particles did not show higher enzyme activity than those without such ingested material (Dannenberg, Walter, and Kapral, 1963). Dannenberg and co-workers have advanced an interesting hypothesis concerning enzyme activation during cellular immunity.

Some of the other enzymes which have been found in alveolar macrophages of various species are listed in the table appearing on pages 48 and 49 of this chapter. It is apparent that the alveolar macrophages of normal animals are constantly subjected to stimuli unique to their environment and that they respond to these stimuli with increased metabolic activity and enzyme synthesis.

3. Blood Monocytes and Tissue Macrophages

Peripheral blood monocytes are relatively immature cells en route to tissue sites where further maturation occurs. Although they may contain a variety of enzymes, the number and size of enzyme-containing lysosomes are characteristically less than those in more mature macrophages found elsewhere.

Macrophages, considered to be derived from blood leukocytes *in vitro* or *in vivo* during inflammation, are similar to histiocytic cells of lymphoid tissue in their enzyme content (cf. review by Elves, 1966). Both macrophages and histiocytic cells of lymphoid tissue are rich in acid phosphatase, 5-nucleotidase, and esterase. It has been proposed that these enzymes reflect cellular function and extent of maturation rather than the identity of macrophage precursors.

Human monocytes from the bone marrow have also been shown to contain lysosomes with peroxidase activity (Dunn, Hardin, and Spicer, 1968).

Gough and Elves (1966, 1967) studied the biochemical constituents and enzyme cytochemistry of lymphocytes, macrophages, and phytohemagglutinin (PHA)-induced blast cells in cultures of the buffy coat of normal human blood. Cultures were maintained for 72 hours in the presence of PHA and examined for blast-cell transformation, or were kept for 48 hours without PHA and observed for lymphocyte-to-macrophage transformation. As compared with unstimulated lymphocytes, PHA-transformed blast cells contained increased amounts of protein, RNA, and sometimes glycogen. The staining characteristics for protein and RNA were reported to be quantitatively the same in the cytoplasm of lymphocytes and macrophages. Some macrophages contained glycogen and fats in blocks within the cytoplasm, suggesting that these materials were derived from ingested PMNs. It was concluded that PHA-stimulated blast transformation of lymphocytes was characterized by greater synthetic activity than was alleged lymphocyte-to-macrophage transformation, and that the changes observed in the macrophages could be the result, at least in part, of their phagocytic activities.

The enzyme content of splenic macrophages is similar to that of macrophages from many other sources. Pettersen (1964) suggested that acid phosphatase and esterase activity are so characteristic of actively phagocytic macrophages as to be a good means of distinguishing these cells from other cells in the rat spleen. Snodgrass (1968) used nonspecific esterase activity and metalophilic properties to classify splenic cells as being reticuloendothelial in nature. Although these enzymes are not restricted to macrophages, within the spleen they are present in appreciable amounts only in macrophages and megakaryocytes.

To recapitulate, in all species studied there is abundant evidence of the presence and synthesis of many enzymes within blood and tissue macrophages, as well as in alveolar and peritoneal macrophages. Some of the lysosomal enzymes which have been demonstrated in macrophages in many locations and in various animals are listed in the table appearing on pages 48 and 49. Although this list is, of necessity, incomplete, it suggests that macrophages can synthesize an unusually wide spectrum of hydrolytic enzymes.

Enzymes Found in Macrophages

Mouse

Peritoneum

      Acid phosphatases (9, 42, 138, 140, 141, 144, 216, 573)
      Acid ribonuclease (138)
      Beta glucuronidase (9, 138, 140, 144, 216, 573)
      Cathepsins (138, 140, 144, 216, 573)
      Esterases (9)

Lung	*Blood*
Acid phosphatases (42)	Acid phosphatases (42)

Liver	*Spleen*
Acid phosphatases (42, 420)	Acid phosphatases (42)

Bone marrow

      Acid phosphatases (42)

Guinea Pig

Peritoneum

Acid phosphatases (381, 512)	Lipases (88, 381)
ATPase (481, 482)	Malic dehydrogenase (512)
Beta glucuronidase (381, 512)	Succinic dehydrogenase (512)
Esterases (381)	

Horse

Blood

Acid phosphatase (45)	BPN hydrolase (45)
Aryl sulfatase (45)	Cytochrome oxidase (45)

Rabbit

Peritoneum

      Acid phosphatases (145, 157, 159, 161, 412, 447)
      Acid ribonucleases (145, 157)
      Aminopeptidase (159)
      Beta glucuronidase (145)
      Cathepsins (145)
      Cytochrome oxidase (159)
      Deoxyribonuclease (157)
      Esterases (121, 145, 157, 158, 159, 161, 175, 180, 412, 447)
      Lipases (121, 145, 157, 158, 412, 447)
      Lysozyme (muramidase) (121, 145, 157, 412, 447, 460)
      Proteases (121, 157, 158, 447)
      Proteinases (412, 447)
      Succinic dehydrogenase (159, 161)

Lung

      Acid phosphatases (145, 157, 159, 161, 310, 399, 447)
      Acid ribonucleases (145, 157)
      Aminopeptidase (159)
      Beta galactosidase (157)
      Beta glucuronidase (145, 157)

Lung (continued)

Beta-N-acetylglucosaminidase (25)
Cathepsins (145, 310)
Cytochrome oxidase (159)
Deoxyribonuclease (157)
Esterases (159, 161, 175, 447)
Lipases (145, 157, 447)
Lysozyme (muramidase) (145, 157, 310, 399, 447, 460, 497)
Proteases (157)
Proteinases (447)
Succinic dehydrogenase (159)

Liver

Esterases (28)

Spleen

Acid phosphatases (597)
Esterases (28, 597)

Epithelioid Cell in Granuloma

Acid phosphatase (160)
Beta galactosidase (160)
Beta glucuronidase (160)
Cytochrome oxidase (160)
Succinic dehydrogenase (160)

Lymph Nodes

Esterases (28)

Rat

Peritoneum

Acid phosphatases (147)
Acid ribonucleases (147)
Beta glucuronidase (147)
Cathepsin (147)

Fructosediphosphate aldolase (147)
Isocitric dehydrogenase (147)
Lysozyme (muramidase) (147)

Spleen

Acid phosphatases (513)
Esterases (513)

Ovary

Acid phosphatases (101)
Beta galactosidase (101)
Esterases (101)

Granuloma Induced by Carrageenan

Galactosidases (449)

Man

Blood

Lipases (88)

Inflammatory Exudate in Skin Window

Acid phosphatases (695)
Alpha glycerophosphate dehydrogenase (692)
DPN- and TPN-diaphorases (692)
Esterases (695)
Isocitric dehydrogenase (693)
Lactic dehydrogenase (693)
Malic dehydrogenase (693)
Succinic dehydrogenase (692)
Uridine diphosphate glucose-glycogen transglycosylase (694)

D. Synthesis of Lipids

It has long been known that macrophages are active in lipid synthesis. For example, Lumb (1954) noted that macrophages consistently participate in the disposal of excess lipids; Byers (1960) reviewed many of the findings which implicate macrophages as being active in lipid synthesis. Included among these findings are evidence for (1) uptake and both hydrolysis and esterification of cholesterol, (2) release of accumulations of cholesterol and vitamin A esters from reticuloendothelial cells after the injection of colloids, (3) uptake of chylomicrons from the serum by cells of the RES in a manner analogous to the uptake of colloids, and (4) a relation between macrophage storage of fats, macrophage proliferation, and the lipidoses (e.g. Hand-Schüller-Christian, Niemann-Pick, Hurler's and Gaucher's diseases).

Antonini (1967) postulated that reduction of the phagocytic functions of the RES in senescence could contribute to the reduced rate of cholesterol metabolism during aging.

Day (1967) reviewed much of the literature on lipid metabolism by macrophages in relation to atherosclerosis. There is much data indicating that macrophages play a major role in both the degradation and synthetic utilization of cholesterol and other lipids.

Macrophages within lymph nodes of the rat readily ingest and retain cholesterol for at least 4 months (French and Morris, 1960). By using either H^3, C^{14}, or P^{32} to label different lipids, Day, Gould-Hurst, Steinborner, and Wahlqvist (1965) showed that, when cholesterol, triglyceride, and phospholipid are ingested simultaneously by lymph node macrophages, cholesterol is removed more slowly than the triglyceride and phospholipid. After the uptake of cholesterol, other lipids accumulate within the lymph nodes, presumably as the result of macrophage metabolism (Day, 1960b). It is possible that cholesterol ester may be utilized by lymph node macrophages in the subsequent synthesis of lipoproteins (Day, Fidge, Gould-Hurst, and Wilkinson, 1965; Day, 1967). Triglycerides are hydrolyzed within lymph node macrophages and the resultant fatty acids are incorporated largely into phospholipid (Day et al., 1966).

Peritoneal and alveolar macrophages may also be active in lipid metabolism. Isolated peritoneal macrophages of the rabbit can incorporate labeled acetate into cholesterol (Day and Fidge, 1964) and can degrade cholesterol. Day and French (1959) and Day (1960a) showed that homogenates of peritoneal macrophages have both synthetic and hydrolytic cholesterol esterase activity. Day and Gould-Hurst (1963) demonstrated partial esterification of C^{14}-labeled cholesterol by homogenates of peritoneal macrophages; the addition of lecithin to the reaction mixture inhibited esterification and facilitated the hydrolysis of cholesterol. Alveolar macrophages have also been shown to contain cholesterol esterase (Day, 1967) and lipase (Cohn and Weiner, 1963; Elsbach, 1965).

Fatty acids and triglycerides are taken up and oxidized by rabbit peritoneal macrophages (Day, 1960c; 1961). By the use of electron microscopy, Casley-Smith and Day (1966) showed that triglyceride emulsions are readily phagocytized by peritoneal macrophages and become localized within large phagosomes. The subsequent appearance of a clear space between the electron-dense triglyceride and the phagosome membrane suggests that the lipid is degraded within the phagosome.

Increased phospholipid synthesis has been reported to accompany high phagocytic activity by peritoneal exudate cells, predominately PMNs (Karnovsky and Wallach, 1961), and probably reflects the formation of many phospholipid phagosomal membranes. Obviously, phagocytic activity by macrophages also demands the formation of new phospholipid membranes. Increased phospholipid synthesis is accompanied by an increase in oxygen uptake and glucose metabolism through the hexose monophosphate shunt (Day, 1967).

It is only remotely possible that the cells that produce lung surfactant are related to alveolar macrophages. Most investigators agree that great alveolar cells produce surfactant. While it has been suggested that these cells can give rise to alveolar macrophages, this suggestion is not widely accepted. Great alveolar cells, also known as type II cells, septal cells, or granular pneumocytes, are the more numerous of the cells which constitute the alveolar wall. By use of the electron microscope and cytochemical techniques, Sorokin (1966) showed that great alveolar cells synthesize and secrete various materials, and that lysosome-like cytosomes of these cells contain considerable amounts of lipids, especially phospholipids. Buckingham et al. (1966) also reported that great alveolar cells synthesize phospholipids, as shown by the incorporation of tritiated acetate or palmitate. Radioautographs of lung revealed that the labeled compounds accumulate within the cytoplasm of the large alveolar cells. The results of Vatter et al. (1968) are in agreement with the concept that type II cells synthesize surfactant and, in addition, showed that the esterase activity of the lung is most prominent in the great alveolar cells. Goldfischer, Kikkawa, and Hoffman (1968) observed that great alveolar cells contain hydrolases and synthesize surfactant; however, these authors do not favor the concept that alveolar macrophages are derived from great alveolar cells. Thus, although it is probable that the great alveolar cell is responsible for the synthesis of surfactant, present evidence provides no substantial support for the concept that it is a precursor of macrophages, and the possible genealogic relationship between this cell and the alveolar macrophage remains undetermined (see also review by Day, 1967).

E. *Synthesis of Interferon*

It is logical to expect that macrophages play an important role in anti-viral defense, especially of the respiratory tract. Recent studies have conclusively demonstrated the production of interferon by macrophages and have established the importance of this cell in defense against viral infections.

Compelling evidence implicating the macrophage as a source of interferon was presented by Kono and Ho (1965), who showed that tissues rich in macrophages, such as spleen and liver, form large quantities of interferon within 24 hours *in vitro*. In contrast, tissues which contain few macrophages, e.g. kidney and brain, formed much smaller quantities of interferon, which were not detectable until after 24 hours. Kono and Ho also measured interferon in the serum of animals given virus 18 hours after a dose of thorium dioxide (Thorotrast) sufficient to cause RES blockade. They noted that in such animals a consistent depression of serum interferon levels was evident at 3 hours after virus inoculation; however, by 7 hours no effect of the thorium dioxide treatment was apparent. It was concluded that reticuloendothelial tissues respond more rapidly to stimuli for interferon production than do other tissues. Moreover, treatment of mice with agents known to cause stimulation of the RES results in the appearance of interferon in the serum, as has been shown by Stinebring and Youngner (1964).

Conclusive evidence that alveolar macrophages can produce interferon has come from the work of Acton and Myrvik (1966). They showed that rabbit alveolar macrophages, inoculated *in vitro* with parainfluenza-3 virus, produce a viral inhibitor which is evidently interferon. The substance is nondialyzable, is stable at pH 4.0, and does not sediment at 100,000 x g. It protects cells of animals of the same species against infection by viruses unrelated to the original virus which induced interferon production. Incubation of normal rabbit alveolar macrophages with this material for 18 hours before challenging the cells with rabbit pox virus protected the cells against destruction by the second virus. Thus, it is clear that alveolar macrophages can produce interferon.

Peritoneal macrophages of rabbits have also been shown to produce interferon (Smith and Wagner, 1967a). These cells synthesized interferon as efficiently as rabbit kidney (RK) cells. By 2 hours after exposure of the macrophages to virus, interferon was detected in the medium and peak titers were found by 4 to 6 hours. Actinomycin blocked interferon production by RK cells if given before 60 to 120 minutes after virus infection and by macrophages only if given prior to 30 to 60 minutes after infection. Smith and Wagner suggested that this may indicate that messenger RNAs responsible for interferon production are transcribed faster and earlier in macrophages than in RK cells.

Smith and Wagner (1967a,b) also showed that bacterial endotoxins and viruses elicit interferon production by rabbit peritoneal macrophages at the same rate. However, the total amount of interferon produced after endotoxin was only 1% or less of that produced in response to virus. The physical properties of the macrophage-produced interferons were examined; the two principal kinds had molecular weights (MWs) of 37,000 and 45,000. In rabbit sera, most interferons have approximate MWs of 51,000 and $>134,000$. The data suggest that interferons produced by peritoneal macrophages are not identical with the majority of serum interferons synthesized in response to viral infection.

F. Synthesis of Serum Proteins

Stecher and Thorbecke (1967a) studied the *in vitro* incorporation of C^{14}-labeled amino acids into serum proteins by various kinds of cells. By use of radioautographic and immunoelectrophoretic techniques they identified labeled serum proteins in cell-free culture fluids. The types of adult rat cells included in the study were thoracic duct cells, peripheral blood leukocytes, and peritoneal exudate cells. The peritoneal cells were separated into fractions rich in either mast cells, eosinophils, or macrophages. It was found that peritoneal macrophages, isolated on glass, synthesized much more β_{1C} globulin (C′ 3) and transferrin than did any of the other cell types. Both peritoneal and alveolar macrophages from mice, guinea pigs, and rabbits invariably produced β_{1C} globulin *in vitro,* whereas primate macrophages synthesized β_{1E} globulin (C′ 4) as well. The synthesis of components of C′ is evidently a common property of macrophages of many mammalian species.

G. Relation of Metabolic Activities to Cellular Functions

The synthetic activities of macrophages, reviewed above, are diverse. As discussed in Chapter 3, it was originally thought that in lower animals the principal function of macrophages was to provide food for the animal by digesting foreign material. During evolution, other functions have become more prominent, a fact reflected, for example, by the capacity of macrophages to synthesize interferon and components of C′, and to degrade foreign and effete autologous cells.

When erythrocytes age and become nonfunctional they are usually destroyed by macrophages (see Chapter 8). Bulmer (1964) described esterase activities in the ovarian macrophages of rats, which he postulated may contribute to the disposal of engulfed erythrocytes, because such macrophages also contain ferric iron, presumably derived from hemoglobin.

Macrophages may normally engulf and degrade effete plasma cells, fibroblasts, and lymphocytes. Swartzendruber (1964) presented electron micrographs which clearly show whole and fragmented plasma cells within tingible-body macrophages of the spleen. *In vitro* studies have shown that effete fibroblasts are disposed of by macrophages (Jacoby, 1965). In special circumstances, e.g. following administration of antilymphocyte serum, lymphocytes that have been injured, killed or opsonized are often observed within macrophages and appear to be in the process of being digested (Pearsall and Weiser, unpublished observation).

After phagocytosis, the lysosomes of macrophages commonly increase both in size and in the intensity of staining for acid phosphatase. The fusion of lysosomes and phagosomes gives rise to large phagolysosomes which react strongly to the test for acid phosphatase, coincident with the disappearance of phagocytized material. Other enzymes, such as esterases, are also demonstrable in the lysosomes early after phagocytosis, and in the phagolysosomes later. It is virtually certain that the activity of these enzymes contributes to the degradation of ingested materials.

There appears to be a relationship between the increased enzyme content of macrophages and cellular immunity. For example, Saito and Suter (1965) and Heise, Myrvik, and Leake (1965) stressed the adaptive capacities of macrophages to respond to stimuli such as BCG infection with an increase in lysosomal enzymes. Similarly, Mizunoe and Dannenberg (1965) suggested that increased levels of hydrolases formed by macrophages *in vivo* in response to tubercle bacilli are probably associated with a high degree of cellular immunity (see Chapter 12).

Carrageenan-induced granulomas in the rat have been used by Monis, Weinberg, and Spector (1968) to study the induction of specific enzymes in macrophages. Carrageenan is a polysaccharide, extracted from Irish moss, composed of a mixture of α and β isomers of sulfated D-polygalactose. Following a single subcutaneous dose of the polysaccharide, granulomatous changes occur. By 7 days there is a marked increase in the number of macrophages in the area, which appears to result from the migration and maturation of blood monocytes and the proliferation of local tissue macrophages. Galactosidases are demonstrable in macrophages which respond to the galactoside-containing carrageenan. By contrast, carrageenan does not contain glucosides and glucosidases are not induced by this substance. This interesting work clearly indicates that a specific induction of macrophage lysosomal enzymes can occur in response to an ingested substrate.

Another point of interest in the work of Monis *et al.* (1968) is that the substance which induced enzyme synthesis is a polysaccharide. Although it is frequently stated that macrophages have little or no capacity to degrade polysaccharides, this is not always true. For example, they often contain lysozyme (muramidase), which hydrolyzes polysaccharide linkages in the aminopolysaccharide, muramic acid. The concept that macrophages cannot degrade polysaccharides probably arose from the observation that substances such as certain pneumococcal polysaccharides are degraded by macrophages poorly or not at all, which may account for the persistence of these polysaccharides in tissues over long periods of time (Kaplan, Coons, and Deane, 1950). It should be appreciated that the ability of macrophages to hydrolyze a given polysaccharide or any other substance, e.g. synthetic polypeptides (Sela, 1966), depends on their genetic potential and on the nature of the chemical linkages in the substance.

The observation of Schwab and Ohanian (1967) that the cell walls of group A streptococci are uniquely resistant to degradation by macrophages is of singular interest. This resistance appears to be correlated with resistance to lysozyme, presumably because the group-specific polysaccharide masks the mucopeptide of the cell wall and protects it from hydrolysis by lysozyme. In consequence, group A streptococcal cell wall materials can persist in tissues and cause chronic irritation.

Enzymic degradation of lipids within macrophages has been clearly demonstrated in some instances (see Section D, above); in other cases it is strongly suggested by morphological appearances. Jacoby (1965) described photographic observations on the disappearance of ingested fats in the living chick macrophage. Several dozen fat granules and droplets, engulfed by one macrophage within an hour, were largely digested when the cell started to divide 3 hours later. Similarly, Tompkins (1946) observed that phagocytized cholesterol disappears from connective tissue macrophages over a period of 5 to 10 days after subcutaneous injection of the substance.

Thus, it is evident that the large quantities of lysosomal hydrolytic enzymes demonstrable within macrophages following phagocytosis are directly concerned in digestion of phagocytized materials, both autologous and foreign. The phagocytosis and processing of potential antigens by macrophages is a topic of particular importance, which will be discussed in Chapter 9, Section A2.

SUMMARY: In general, macrophages exhibit a high degree of metabolic activity. Their metabolic requirements *in vitro* have not been well defined. Usually serum is required for their cultivation, and an undefined growth factor obtained from syngeneic or allogeneic fibroblast cultures can stimulate metabolism and proliferation *in vitro*.

Macrophages contain the enzymes needed for a variety of energy-yielding metabolic pathways. Whereas peritoneal macrophages obtain energy principally through glycolysis, alveolar macrophages rely largely on oxidative metabolism for their energy. The hexose monophosphate shunt is a major source of energy for the increased metabolism of alveolar macrophages during periods of cellular activity.

In addition to the enzymes concerned with energy production, macrophages synthesize a wide variety of lysosomal hydrolytic enzymes which function in the digestion of phagocytized materials. They are capable of synthesizing interferon and serum proteins, including certain components of complement. They also contain enzymes for the synthesis and degradation of lipids.

The extensive synthetic activities of macrophages clearly contribute to their marked capacities to degrade ingested materials, to participate in iron metabolism, to afford protection against invasion by foreign agents such as bacteria and viruses, and to provide essential substances such as phospholipids and components of complement.

Chapter 7

Phagocytosis by Macrophages

PHAGOCYTIC CAPABILITY is a basic property of macrophages; although macrophages may not exhibit this ability at all times, they must, by definition, be potentially capable of phagocytosis. The biological and physicochemical sequences leading to the engulfment of particulates have been studied most extensively in PMNs; nevertheless, much information is also available concerning phagocytosis by macrophages. Many facts about phagocytosis have been learned from studies of other kinds of mammalian cells, and of amebae.

A. *Uptake of Extracellular Materials by Macrophages*

Macrophages take up materials by phagocytosis and in other ways. Phagocytosis is defined as the engulfment by cells of particulates large enough to be readily visible by light microscopy. Pinocytosis, sometimes called microphagocytosis, is a similar process by which soluble materials or particles of submicroscopic size are ingested. Cohn and co-workers have conducted extensive studies on pinocytosis by macrophages (Cohn and Benson, 1965c; Cohn, 1966; and Cohn and Parks, 1967a, b, c).

Pinocytosis means, literally, drinking by the cell. During this process, extracellular material is trapped in vesicles formed by invagination of the cell membrane (cf. reviews by Holter, 1959a, b; Chapman-Andresen, 1962). In the macrophage, pinocytic vesicles are frequently 1 to 2 μ in diameter; however, they vary in size considerably. These vesicles pinch off from the cell membrane and migrate toward the nucleus. Cohn, Fedorko, and Hirsch (1966) described the uptake of colloidal gold in micropinocytic vesicles, a number of which subsequently fused to form large pinosomes which in turn fused with lysosomes. Presumably the pinocytosis of metabolizable materials and their subsequent exposure to hydrolytic enzymes allows their breakdown and utilization by the macrophage.

Pinocytosis can be induced in cultured mouse macrophages by the addition of high molecular weight anions (Cohn and Parks, 1967a). It is a discontinuous process, at least *in vitro*. Macrophages are actively pinocytic for a time after being placed in culture; then pinocytosis ceases until fresh medium is added (Jacoby, 1965). Many substances, including anti-

Phagocytosis requires energy (see next section), in addition to being temperature-dependent. It is decreased as the temperature decreases, below the optimum (37° C to 42° C for mammalian phagocytes). Although phagocytosis of bacteria and yeast by rabbit peritoneal macrophages occurs within a pH range from 2.5 to 10.0, the optimum pH is between 7.0 and 8.5 (Tucker, Hill, and Gifford, 1963). Similar findings have been reported for human monocytes by Cline and Lehrer (1968).

Berry and Spies (1949) reviewed the physicochemical aspects of phago-cytosis. The properties of macrophage plasma membranes which encourage their characteristic penchant for phagocytosis are not well defined; how-ever, several of their properties may contribute. The ability of macrophages to actively synthesize and degrade a variety of lipids could be related to the capacity of macrophages to maintain the rapid turnover of phospho-lipid cell membranes required during phagocytosis and pinocytosis (Kar-novsky and Wallach, 1961; Cohn, 1966; Elsbach, 1968). In addition, cytophilic antibodies for macrophages facilitate the adherence of particu-lates to the cell and thus promote particle engulfment. This could apply not only to the material for which the cytophilic antibodies are specific, but also in a more limited way to unrelated substances which may be bound or attracted nonspecifically to globulins.

A method for accurate measurement of phagocytosis by macrophages has been described by Carpenter and Barsales (1967), who used bentonite particles of an appropriate size coated with I^{125}-labeled protein. The pro-tein was stabilized by reaction with carbodiimide to limit its release from the suspended bentonite. It was found that cultured macrophages from guinea pig spleen generally require opsonins for phagocytosis, and that these opsonins consist of heat-labile nonspecific factors in nonimmune serum and heat-stable specific antibodies in immune serum. Presumably the heat-labile factors are components of C'.

The morphology and function of cells of respiratory tissues of numerous animal species has been reviewed by Bertalanffy (1964), who showed that alveolar cells phagocytized material within 4 minutes after its intratracheal introduction, and the peak of phagocytic activity occurred 6 to 16 minutes later. The ameboid movement of these alveolar cells was typical of macrophages, as described in Chapter 2. The many lipid droplets observed in over half of the phagocytic cells may have represented an accumulation of lipids derived from blood passing through lung capillaries. Approxi-mately 20% of the alveolar cells from rats phagocytized carbon during 30 minutes *in vitro*.

To recapitulate, macrophages from various sources phagocytize particles by a two-stage mechanism. The first stage consists of contact of the particle with the cell, as a result of chance encounter, chemotactic attrac-tion, or antibody activity. The second stage, consisting of actual ingestion of the particle, is energy-dependent and requires divalent cations and serum factors. These requirements could explain, at least in part, why not all macrophages are actively phagocytic even though they are endowed with phagocytic capability.

C. Phagocytic Energy Requirements

The biochemical aspects of the energy-requiring phagocytic process have been reviewed by Karnovsky (1962). Karnovsky (1961) also summarized the metabolic shifts which occur during phagocytosis. He and his colleagues used monocytes or PMNs from peritoneal exudates, suspended in medium containing a C^{14}-labeled energy source. Both the disposition of C^{14} and the oxygen uptake were determined at rest or during phagocytosis. Inert particles such as polystyrene were often used to measure the extent of phagocytosis since serum is not required for efficient engulfment of these particles. It was found that peritoneal monocytes increased their oxygen uptake approximately threefold during phagocytosis. Differences between metabolic patterns in actively phagocytic macrophages and PMNs were noted.

Oren *et al.* (1963) reported that oxygen uptake of resting guinea pig peritoneal macrophages is approximately three times that of PMNs and only one fourth that of resting alveolar macrophages. During phagocytosis, respiration increases to 2.5 times normal in PMNs, 3.5 times normal in peritoneal macrophages, and to only some 20% above normal in alveolar macrophages. Exposure to the glycolysis inhibitors, iodoacetate and fluoride, inhibits the phagocytic activity of alveolar and peritoneal macrophages, as well as PMNs. Inhibition of oxidative metabolism, by anaerobiosis, dinitrophenol, or cyanide, suppresses phagocytosis by alveolar macrophages but not by PMNs or peritoneal macrophages, showing that alveolar macrophages depend on aerobic oxidative metabolism for energy needs in phagocytosis.

Myrvik and Evans (1967a,b) have demonstrated increased metabolism via the hexose monophosphate shunt by alveolar macrophages which were actively phagocytic.

It has been shown that iodoacetate or fluoride inhibits phagocytosis by guinea pig splenic macrophages (Carpenter and Barsales, 1967) and by human monocytes (Cline and Lehrer, 1968), suggesting the necessity of glycolysis as an energy source for phagocytosis by these cells.

Newly formed macrophages in the liver are not actively phagocytic (Rubin, 1964), perhaps because they require time to generate the energy needed for phagocytosis.

North (1966a) used histochemical staining in conjunction with electron microscopy to show that the cytoplasmic membranes of guinea pig peritoneal macrophages contain adenosine triphosphatase (ATPase). The enzyme was active in the presence of the divalent cations, Ca^{++} and Mg^{++}, and was inhibited by sulfhydryl poisons, by adenosine diphosphate, or by treatment of the cells for 30 minutes with 0.5% trypsin. North suggested that this membrane-bound ATPase acts as an energy source for phagocytosis by peritoneal macrophages.

North (1968) also studied the cellular activity of macrophages during spreading on a surface. It was assumed that spreading represents an attempt by the cell to phagocytize the surface. North showed that ATP is a limiting factor in both spreading and phagocytosis and suggested that opsonins may enhance phagocytosis by initiating cell-surface enzymatic reactions which induce the synthesis of more ATP.

D. The Role of Humoral Factors in Phagocytosis

Serum is necessary for the efficient phagocytosis of most particles (Howard and Wardlaw, 1958; Wardlaw and Howard, 1959; Rowley, 1962; North, 1968). The suggestion has been made that opsonins must always be present in order for phagocytosis to occur. Nonspecific opsonins, which are capable of opsonizing a wide variety of particulates, may exist. Fibrin has been proposed as an agent that may nonspecifically opsonize particles under certain circumstances (Wilkins, 1967). It has long been appreciated that the presence of specific opsonins in immune serum greatly increases the rate of phagocytosis by macrophages and PMNs (Berry and Spies, 1949). In fact, certain virulent organisms (e.g. capsulated type III pneumococci) may even escape surface phagocytosis unless specific opsonins are present. Stuart (1967) presented evidence suggesting that the ability of human macrophages to discriminate between RBCs of various human blood groups and of different species depends on opsonins.

Rabinovitch (1968) reported that the attachment of glutaraldehyde-treated erythrocytes (GRCs) to mouse peritoneal macrophages in serum-free medium was decreased if the macrophages were trypsinized. However, specific anti-erythrocyte serum facilitated the attachment of GRCs to either the trypsinized or non-trypsinized macrophages. These results suggest that different receptor sites may exist on peritoneal macrophages, some effective for GRCs and others for antibody-coated erythrocytes. In addition, there is evidence that the receptors on macrophages from different strains of mice differ (Perkins et al., 1967). It is also known that macrophages bear a variety of receptors for different classes of antibodies (see Chapter 10). Thus the class and amount of antibody present may strongly influence the rate and extent of phagocytosis.

Complement plays a major role in phagocytosis (see reviews by Austen and Cohn, 1963; Müller-Eberhard, 1968). When components of C′ aggregate with antibody to form the complex C′1,4,2,3, phagocytosis is enhanced. Natural antibodies, i.e. antibodies which are formed without deliberate exposure to antigens, are commonly present in nonimmune sera and often promote phagocytosis by generating formation of the C' complex. Agglutinins can aggregate bacteria and cause the formation of antigen: antibody:C' complexes which are avidly phagocytized. In immune sera, containing specific antibodies, phagocytosis of gram-positive bacteria is markedly enhanced by the combined activity of opsonins and C'. Antibodies against surface antigens of certain gram-negative bacilli (e.g. *Escherichia coli, Salmonella typhosa*) are bacteriolytic when C' is present, thus obviating phagocytosis. In the absence of C', however, these antibodies may also aid in promoting phagocytosis.

The phagocytosis-promotion factors (PPF) which have been described in normal serum (Tullis and Surgenor, 1956) are alleged to be independent of C'. Their nature has not been determined.

Bosworth and Archer (1962) described a different phagocytosis-promoting substance present in eosinophils. Particles coated with this substance were readily phagocytized by peritoneal macrophages.

Other evidence indicating that serum components contribute to phagocytosis by the RES has come from the work of Normann and Benditt (1965b). The factor described by these investigators is an unidentified protein which can be concentrated by adsorption to and subsequent elution from barium sulfate or other materials. An analogous factor was found in rat, rabbit, hog, and human sera.

Vaughan (1965) demonstrated that phagocytosis of foreign particles by rabbit peritoneal macrophages depends on specific natural opsonic antibodies present in rabbit serum, which account for discriminative phagocytosis by these cells. The opsonins can be demonstrated on well-washed macrophages, and hence must be cytophilic.

Cohn and Parks (1967c) investigated pinocytosis by mouse macrophages, which was induced *in vitro* by incubation in high concentrations of serum. It was found that newborn or adult bovine serum contains a natural antibody which is cytotoxic for RBCs and macrophages of mice. In the absence of C', this antibody stimulated the membranes of macrophages, resulting in intense pinocytic activity. Continuous exposure of macrophages to this specific globulin led to extensive turnover of cell membrane, during which much of the existing cytoplasmic membrane was used to form pinocytic vesicles and new exterior membrane was synthesized. This antibody, in common with other inducers of pinocytosis, caused a marked increase in the number of lysosomes containing hydrolytic enzymes.

Thus it is apparent that serum factors are essential for optimal phagocytosis. Included among the serum components known to facilitate phagocytosis are the following: natural antibodies, immune antibodies, and C' complexes.

E. *Reticuloendothelial Functions*

Phagocytosis and clearance of foreign particles from the circulation are prime functions of the RES. Consequently they have received a major share of research attention, and there is a vast literature on the subject. Only the briefest discussion of RES clearance is possible here; however, references to some of the available reviews and publications are presented.

Measurement of RES clearance is complicated by the fact that there is no consensus as to what cells constitute the system; however, there is general agreement that macrophages are a major component of the RES (Baillif, 1960; Snell, 1960; Cohn, 1965). Heller (1958) reviewed the early literature on the measurement of RES clearance. The general practice is to inject inert colloids intravenously (i.v.) and follow their clearance from the blood stream. The colloids must, in addition to being inert, have a uniform particle size and must not aggregate spontaneously either *in vitro* or *in vivo*. Carbon stabilized with gelatin has been widely used, as have latex, polystyrene, thorium dioxide, and numerous other particulates. Following injection, the rate of removal of particles from the blood is exponential. Heller (1958) presented a characteristic graph which shows a straight line relationship between the optical density (as a measure of particles remaining in the circulation) and the elapsed time in minutes following i.v. injection of a suitable dose of carbon into mice. The graph shows that 50% of the carbon was removed from the circulation in 20 minutes.

Fred and Shore (1967) described a more complex mathematical model for RES function. Their work suggests that phagocytosis involves a rate-limiting interaction between the macrophage surface and the particle being ingested.

Other techniques, reviewed by Heller (1958), involve the intravenous injection of radioactively labeled particles, either bacteria or compounds in colloidal suspension. The disappearance of radioactivity from the blood stream provides a measure of RES clearance. Singer and co-workers (1967) used radioiodinated latex particles for studies of phagocytosis.

A temporary blockade of the RES can be achieved by depleting essential serum factors and perhaps by overloading the cells so that they can no longer take up the test colloid. By use of *in vitro* liver perfusion, or a double perfusion system, Jeunet and co-workers (Jeunet and Good, 1967; 1969; Jeunet, Cain, and Good, 1969) studied the mechanisms of RES clearance. Their evidence indicates that RES blockade may result from two effects, acting separately or together, i.e. a depletion of humoral opsonic factors and/or a cellular blockade. They suggested that the cellular blockade may be due to exhaustion of membrane receptor sites concerned with the phagocytosis of specific compounds or chemically related substances.

It is probable that macrophages usually do not become overloaded with particles, since in many instances of blockade the cells are still capable of phagocytizing other kinds of particulates. Rather, it seems likely that exhaustion of serum opsonins (Pisano, Patterson, and DiLuzio, 1968) or of receptor sites on the cells (Fred and Shore, 1967) accounts for the temporary blockade.

Because cells of the RES can increase in numbers rapidly, blockade is a transient condition and compensatory proliferation soon leads to increased clearance rates (Biozzi *et al.,* 1956). Substances such as silica or thorium dioxide, which destroy macrophages, would be expected to cause a recovery rate different from that observed following blockade with carbon or other inert substances. In addition, the marked capacity of macrophages to synthesize new membranes could defeat attempts at long-lasting blockade.

F. Additional Factors Known to Influence Phagocytosis and Reticuloendothelial Functions

Simultaneous exposure of RES cells to more than one kind of particle can influence the rate of phagocytosis. For example, Normann and Benditt (1965a) found that either heat-aggregated albumin or foreign red cells inhibited carbon clearance when given simultaneously with the carbon. They attributed this effect to depletion of serum factors (Normann and Benditt, 1965b). Using a different experimental system, Rabinovitch and Gary (1968) demonstrated that mouse peritoneal macrophages become activated following the phagocytosis of staphylococci and ingest more GRCs than nonstimulated macrophages. Evidently this was due to an increase in the proportion of macrophages ingesting GRCs, rather than to a more efficient uptake per macrophage. The report of Dobson, Kelly, and Finney (1967) that repeated injections of carbon led to increased clearance rates, rather than to RES blockade, could rest on activation of existing macrophages.

It is especially noteworthy that phagocytosis of one kind of particle may commit the macrophage to metabolic activities concerned with the degradation of that particle, to the exclusion of other possible functions. For example, patients with sickle cell anemia and certain other hemolytic disorders are highly susceptible to salmonella infections. Prompted by this clinical observation, Gill, Kaye, and Hook (1966) and Kaye, Gill, and Hook (1967) showed, in animal studies, that extensive erythrophagocytosis interferes with the capacity of macrophages to kill antibody-coated salmonellae which are subsequently ingested.

Perkins and Leonard (1963) made the interesting observation that the percent of foreign RBCs engulfed by mouse peritoneal macrophages, in the presence or absence of serum opsonins, is directly proportional to the genetic disparity between the phagocytes and the RBCs. This suggests that cytophilic antibodies on macrophages might contribute to phagocytosis, since natural antibodies of more specificities would be present when the RBCs are more antigenically disparate.

Thus the evidence cited above indicates that opsonins, either in the serum or cell-bound, are essential for phagocytosis. These opsonins may be antibodies highly specific for the antigens of the particles; they may be relatively nonspecific opsonic factors, or even totally nonspecific. After macrophages have become activated by ingestion of one type of particle they may be able to phagocytize other particles more readily because of increased metabolic activity. It is possible that, following extensive phagocytosis of one kind of particle, the available mature, functional lysosomes are expended, hence lysosomal enzymes are not available for the digestion of particles that are subsequently phagocytized. Alternatively the macrophage may be committed to the production of enzymes necessary for the degradation of the first kind of particles and may be unable to produce those needed to destroy the second kind.

The importance of hormonal influences on RES function is well established. Gordon and Katsh (1949) concluded that the adrenal cortex is important in the regulation of RES activity. Thorium dioxide (ThO_2) was employed as the i.v. test agent and chemical analysis for thorium was used to measure ThO_2 content of the spleen. It was found that adrenalectomy results in decreased ThO_2 uptake by the spleen, and that administration of whole adrenal cortical extract increases uptake in adrenalectomized rats. Hypophysectomy did not affect the removal of circulating ThO_2 by the rat spleen; nevertheless, when large amounts of adrenal cortical extract were given to hypophysectomized rats, a marked increase in the uptake of ThO_2 occurred.

The effects of cortisone on macrophage function were also investigated by Gell and Hinde (1953), who studied the uptake of colloidal gold within 4 minutes after its intravenous administration, and the uptake of killed staphylococci in the peritoneum during 10 minutes after their injection. At these early post-injection intervals there was no significant difference between the cortisone-treated and control animals. Gell and Hinde suggested that cortisone acts on the RES by altering the tissue environment and suppressing cell mobility. Others (Spain, Molomut, and Haber, 1950) concluded that cortisone inhibits phagocytic function either by decreasing the activity of individual cells or by inhibiting the mobilization of cells. In Spain, Molomut, and Haber's experiments, mobility of macrophages was essential to the removal of injected carbon, and lack of phagocyte mobility, rather than inhibition of actual phagocytosis, could have accounted for the delayed clearance.

Low concentrations of corticosteroids have been reported by Snell (1960) to stimulate phagocytosis by the RES in mice. Cortisone and hydrocortisone (<5 mg/kg) produced an increased rate of blood clearance of chromium phosphate, which lasted longer than 24 hours. Conversely, a high dose (250 mg/kg) of the steroids caused RES blockade. Similar results were obtained by Nicol and Bilbey (1958), indicating that dosage and timing of drug administration are of primary importance in effecting either stimulation or depression of RES function.

Hormones other than those of the adrenal and hypophysis may influence RES activity. For example, it has been shown that thyroid hormone affects the disposition of particulate matter by macrophages. Lurie (1960) and others (see Chapter 12, Section B) reported that hyperthyroidism increases the native resistance of rabbits to tuberculosis by increasing macrophage activity. In hyperthyroid rabbits, phagocytes with ingested tubercle bacilli matured more rapidly into epithelioid cells than did similar cells of animals with normal thyroid function. Conversely, thyroidectomy or cortisone treatment of the rabbits resulted in depressed macrophage function and decreased resistance to tuberculosis.

Nicol, Bilbey, and Ware (1958), Bilbey and Nicol (1963), and Nicol, Vernon-Roberts, and Quantock (1966) demonstrated that estrogens can stimulate RES activity, and that estrogenicity and RES-stimulating activity may reside in different parts of the hormone molecule. The stimulating effects of estrogens on RES activity were also studied by Flemming (1967).

Stimulation of RES function can be achieved in many other ways. Simple triglycerides stimulate phagocytic activity (Cooper and West, 1962; Stuart, 1963; Cooper, 1964), perhaps by activating the macrophages (Carr and Williams, 1967). Other nontoxic RES-stimulatory lipids from yeasts and sharks, called restim, have been described by Heller (1960), Ransom, Pasternak, and Heller (1962), and Heller, Ransom, and Pasternak (1963). Still other agents or circumstances that can stimulate phagocytosis and RES clearance include histamine and 5-hydroxytryptamine (Northover, 1961; Fernex, 1968), infecting bacteria, bacterial extracts (Halpern, Biozzi, and Stiffel, 1963), neoplasms (Old *et al.,* 1960), graft-versus-host reactions (Boak *et al.,* 1968), and allograft reactions (Fisher and Fisher, 1964).

Depression of RES function can be caused by alkyl esters of fatty acids such as methyl or ethyl palmitate (Stuart, 1963; Blickens and DiLuzio, 1965; Flemming, 1967; Saba and DiLuzio, 1968). Nicol and Bilbey (1958) tabulated a number of substances which depress RES phagocytosis. The strong depressants included cortisone acetate, prednisone, prednisolone, and 4-hyroxytetraphenylmethane; the mild depressants included ergosterol, lanosterol, cholesterol, and stilbene.

Bacterial endotoxins can either stimulate or depress RES function, depending on a number of factors such as dosage and schedule of administration. The extremely diverse effects of endotoxins have stimulated an immense amount of investigation into the nature and possible mechanisms of action of these substances. An excellent source of references on the chemistry and biological effects of endotoxins is provided by the symposium proceedings edited by Landy and Braun (1964).

Bacterial endotoxins are complex mixtures of lipopolysaccharides produced by any of a variety of gram-negative bacteria. However, the biological effects of these different endotoxins are remarkably similar, and include pyrogenicity, leukopenia followed by leukocytosis, platelet abnormalities, hemorrhagic lesions in viscera and skin, endocrine stimulation with release of endogenous adrenocorticotropic hormone, and metabolic changes (Bennett and Cluff, 1957). Endotoxins could affect RES function by virtue of their toxicity, some other direct activity of the molecules, some indirect action such as endocrine stimulation, or a combination of these factors. Direct cytotoxic action is almost certainly implicated, since macrophages *in vitro* (isolated from endocrine and other influences) are very sensitive to the cytotoxic effects of endotoxins (Heilman, 1963, 1964, 1965; Kessel and Braun, 1965). On the other hand, macrophages can detoxify endotoxins both *in vitro* (Rutenburg, Schweinburg, and Fine, 1960) and *in vivo* (Wiznitzer *et al.,* 1960), as discussed in Chapter 8, Section C-1. Obviously the mechanisms leading to RES activation or depression by endotoxins are complex and poorly understood.

The effects of x-irradiation on cells of the RES have been studied by a number of investigators. As early as 1935, Chrom reported that, whereas injected bacteria were completely cleared from the circulation of normal mice in 12 to 15 hours, they were not cleared from the circulation of x-irradiated mice within 72 hours. However, when the liver and spleen were shielded during x-irradiation, the bacilli were cleared within 16 hours. Chrom concluded that cells of the RES become functionally impaired by x-irradiation.

There is general agreement that RES cells show no morphological evidence of damage following x-irradiation (Bloom, 1948; Brecher *et al.,* 1948). The data concerning RES function are not so clear-cut; conflicting reports have appeared concerning the rate of clearance of intravenously injected substances from the circulation of irradiated animals. Barrow, Tullis, and Chambers (1951) studied the effect of x-irradiation on clearance of colloidal radiogold injected i.v. into rabbits. The clearance rates varied markedly among control rabbits, and were not altered by doses of 500 r or 800 r of x ray. Thorotrast (ThO$_2$), on the other hand, suppressed clearance almost completely when given 16 hours prior to the gold. Treatment with ThO$_2$ 18 hours prior to administration of the gold caused a prolonged clearance time, indicating that recovery from the temporary RES blockade was occurring. The ability of macrophages in organ cultures to segregate carmine was not impaired by *in vitro* doses of x ray as high as 40 kr to 100 kr (Gilman and Trowell, 1965).

Gabrieli and Auskaps (1953) obtained similar results with different doses of x ray given to rats. Chromium phosphate was cleared at the normal rate over a 4-week period following doses of 25 r to 100 r of x ray; however, the organ distribution of the phagocytized material was different from that observed in nonirradiated rats. DiLuzio (1955) reported comparable findings, using a high dose of x ray and radioactive colloidal gold as the test substance, as did Benacerraf et al. (1959) using either colloidal particles or P^{32}-labeled Escherichia coli. The conclusion which can be drawn from these and similar experiments is that the phagocytic capacity of macrophages is unaltered by sublethal doses of x ray, even though vascular permeability changes and other factors may alter the distribution of phagocytized materials in organs.

Although bacteria and foreign erythrocytes are cleared from the circulation of x-irradiated animals at the normal rate for a time after injection, there is evidence that cells of the RES cannot retain and degrade these substances in a normal manner (Gordon, Cooper, and Miller, 1955; Donaldson and co-workers, 1956). The effect of x-irradiation on intracellular degradation of phagocytized material will be discussed with respect to antibody synthesis in Chapter 9.

SUMMARY: Macrophages take up extracellular materials by phagocytosis, pinocytosis, and similar processes. Phagocytosis occurs in two stages, attachment and ingestion. During the first phase, particles attach to the cell as a result of a chance encounter, chemotactic attraction, or antibody activity. The second phase, ingestion, is energy-dependent and requires divalent cations and serum factors.

Phagocytosis is temperature-dependent, with optimum temperatures of 37° C to 42° C for mammalian macrophages. The optimum pH range is between 7.0 and 8.5; however, phagocytosis can occur within a pH range from 2.5 to 10.0. The energy source for phagocytosis by macrophages is largely glycolysis, which may be supplemented by aerobic respiration to varying degrees, or by energy-yielding enzyme reactions at the cell surface.

Serum factors which facilitate phagocytosis include antibodies, complement, and several other less well-defined components. The extent and rate of phagocytosis by macrophages of the RES are frequently measured by quantitating the clearance of injected substance from the blood stream. Additional factors which are known to influence phagocytosis and other functions of the RES include: simultaneous exposure of RES cells to more than one kind of particle; hormone activities; lipids; endotoxins; x-irradiation; bacterial infections; tumor growth; and certain cellular immunological reactions.

Chapter 8

Functions of Macrophages

MACROPHAGES have many important functions. They act as scavengers to dispose of foreign matter and effete autologous cells; most ingested substances are degraded and many of the products are utilized in body economy. In addition, macrophages play an important role in immunological events, and have a number of other specialized functions.

A. Scavenger Activities

Some of the mechanisms involved in the clearance of foreign and effete material from the circulation have been discussed previously. The foreign material commonly disposed of by macrophages includes bacteria and many kinds of inhaled or injected substances, both particulate and soluble.

1. Cytophilic Opsonins as an Aid in Scavenger Activities

Enhancement of the phagocytic activities of macrophages by specific opsonins has been well documented (see Chapter 7, Section D). Many opsonins act by coating particles and changing their surfaces, either by altering surface charges or in other ways. In theory, such a mechanism might require extensive coating of surfaces by antibody and would prepare the particles for engulfment by all types of phagocytes. However, many opsonins are cytophilic for macrophages (Berken and Benacerraf, 1966). A portion of the cytophilic antibody molecule, distinct from its antigen-combining sites, can bind weakly but specifically with receptors on the macrophage membrane (see Chapter 10). Specific attachment of particles to the phagocyte surface occurs if the cytophilic antibody is first attached to the macrophage and then combines with antigen, or if antigen and antibody combine before cytophilic attachment is achieved. In either case, little cytophilic antibody may be required for the attachment of particles and their subsequent engulfment by the macrophage. When the particles are cells with few antigenic sites on their surfaces, complete engulfment may not occur; instead, phagocytic action may be limited to "membrane phagocytosis" in which small bits of the membrane of opsonized cells are phagocytized by macrophages. Usually, the close association between opsonized particle and macrophage membrane afforded by the cytophilic attachment greatly facilitates phagocytosis. In addition, the influx of macrophages into sites of scavenger activity, such as areas of infection, provides a means for carrying opsonins attached to cytophilic receptors directly to the point where they are needed. Cytophilic antibodies on macrophages throughout the body contribute to a surveillance mechanism which functions to utilize small amounts of antibody most effectively.

Although many types of cells have limited phagocytic capabilities, specific opsonins appear to promote the uptake of particles only by strongly phagocytic cells such as macrophages and PMNs (North, 1968). Perhaps these are the only cells with receptors for cytophilic opsonins, either free or combined with antigen.

The contribution of cytophilic antibodies to the destruction of effete autologous erythrocytes by macrophages is not defined. Apparently opsonins are not required for the adherence to macrophages of RBCs altered by storage (Vaughan and Boyden, 1964). However, the second phase of phagocytosis, during which ingestion of adhering particles occurs, may require opsonic action. Jenkin and Karthigasu (1962) suggested that opsonins are necessary for the removal of effete RBCs by macrophages. Since the first phase of phagocytosis, adherence, does not require energy or divalent cations, whereas the second phase does, it is probable that opsonins are essential for only the ingestion phase of phagocytosis of effete erythrocytes, but facilitate both phases.

2. Disposal of Tissue Debris and Effete Cells

One of the major functions of macrophages is to dispose of tissue debris and effete cells. Macrophages, and not PMNs, are responsible for the removal of autochthonous materials. Vaughan (1965) observed that this activity is not attributable to serum antibodies. This does not rule out the possibility that cytophilic antibodies on macrophages can recognize materials which have become "foreign" because of antigenic changes during aging. Although some extraneous materials may be nonmetabolizable, ingested cellular constituents are usually readily metabolized. Thus the conservation and reutilization of cellular components, e.g. iron compounds, are facilitated by macrophage activities.

The role of the macrophage in iron metabolism is well established. Ingested iron compounds are absorbed by mucosal cells of the intestine and the iron is incorporated into ferritin. In the presence of reducing agents the iron is freed from the ferritin molecules and is bound to the β_1 globulin of the serum, transferrin. Each molecule of this protein has two binding sites for iron (Wintrobe, 1961). The iron is tightly bound by transferrin and delivered directly to erythroblasts in the bone marrow or to other cells concerned with iron metabolism (Bessis, 1963). Transferrin binds specifically to receptors on the surfaces of certain cells and may deliver one atom of iron to the erythroblast and retain the other one, eventually storing it in the liver or elsewhere. Thus, transferrin is responsible for the distribution of iron throughout the body (Fletcher and Huehns, 1968). When iron is injected subcutaneously, its ingestion and the subsequent synthesis of ferritin in the macrophage cytoplasm can be studied by electron microscopy. Muir and Golberg (1961) described the pinocytic ingestion of iron-dextran by macrophages, the subsequent synthesis of apoferritin, and the incorporation of iron into ferritin molecules. Normally, excess iron is carried to the liver, where it is stored as ferritin (Thompson, 1961). Numerous ferritin granules are also seen in the cytoplasm of free alveolar macrophages (Karrer, 1960).

Although many substances are cleared from the blood stream largely by Kupffer cells of the liver, macrophages in the spleen and bone marrow account for most of the removal of effete nonsensitized erythrocytes. Within the macrophage, part of the hemoglobin is transformed to bilirubin which is eliminated via the liver, and iron and globin are retained and utilized (Dacie, 1960).

Macrophages which transport and store iron are not found in the blood of normal human subjects; however, Yam and co-workers (1968) found circulating iron-containing macrophages in a considerable percentage of patients with iron-storage diseases. Such cells were found rarely in patients with extreme iron-loading. In hemochromatosis, macrophages contain smaller granules of iron than in transfusion siderosis.

Erythrophagocytosis by macrophages can be seen in tissues from healthy individuals, but Essner (1960) has reviewed the evidence suggesting that phagocytosis does not occur often enough to account for the normal rate of destruction of RBCs. Of more importance is the process of fragmentation of erythrocytes, during which portions of the cells are pinched off and are subsequently ingested by macrophages. Doan and Sabin (1926) observed fragmentation of rabbit erythrocytes. Their interpretation was that poikilocytes represent the first stage of fragmentation and that microcytes result from loss of part of the red cell. Fragmentation was found to be constant in normal animals, and was greatly increased in various types of anemias.

The adherence of effete RBCs to macrophages, which can occur even in the absence of opsonins (Vaughan and Boyden, 1964), would allow effective membrane phagocytosis to occur. Therefore, the processes of fragmentation and membrane phagocytosis may account for much of the disposal of nonsensitized, as well as antibody-sensitized, erythrocytes (Rous, 1923; Weed and Reed, 1966).

Thus, macrophages not only serve as scavengers in the normal destruction of effete erythrocytes, but also function to conserve the iron present in these cells by their metabolic, transport, and storage activities.

There is abundant evidence that effete cells other than erythrocytes are phagocytized and metabolized by macrophages. For example, plasma cells and plasma cell fragments have been identified within tingible-body macrophages of the spleen (Swartzendruber, 1964). Myelin bodies and other materials frequently seen in the cytoplasm of macrophages provide additional evidence that effete cells are being disposed of by these phagocytes.

The many macrophages in the thymus undoubtedly serve to remove debris resulting from the rapid turnover of cells in this organ. Kostowiecki (1963) has reviewed the literature on thymic macrophages.

It is well established that macrophages play a major role in the resorption of tissue following inflammation, and in certain physiological circumstances. For example, Mayberry (1964) and Helminen and Ericsson (1968a, b, c) described the activities of macrophages in post-secretory mammary involution, and Deno (1937) reported an interesting study of their activities during postpartum involution of the mouse uterus. Whereas PMNs were the cells most active in removing debris during the first 2 days of the puerperium, macrophages subsequently assumed the major role of phagocytizing and digesting effete cells and cell remnants. The macrophages became filled with hemosiderin derived from erythrocyte digestion, and aggregated to form brown areas grossly visible on the dorsal surface of the uterus.

The reutilization of resorbed materials, as well as foreign substances, is accomplished by macrophages. Ehrenreich and Cohn (1968a, b) followed the fate of ingested proteins within mouse peritoneal macrophages. After their pinocytosis, radioactively labeled proteins were digested to the level of amino acids, or possibly small peptides and amino acids. It was postulated that pinocytosis by macrophages may make a considerable contribution toward the turnover of serum proteins, the conservation of stores of iron, cellular nutrition, and other metabolic events.

3. Action of Macrophages on Sensitized Erythrocytes

The fate of RBCs which have been sensitized by exposure to specific antibodies, either *in vitro* or *in vivo,* differs in several respects from that of nonsensitized effete cells. Whereas red cells are normally removed largely by macrophages in the spleen and bone marrow, sensitized erythrocytes are frequently eliminated from the circulation within the liver and other organs. Sabin and Doan (1926) and Doan and Sabin (1926) studied RBC destruction in tuberculous rabbits. Macrophages loaded with red cell fragments were found in the lungs, as well as in the spleen and bone marrow. In some cases the macrophages from these rabbits had erythrocytes adhering to them.

A similar red cell-macrophage adherence is shown in the electron micrographs of LoBuglio, Cotran, and Jandl (1967). These investigators reported that macrophages rapidly remove sensitized erythrocytes from the blood stream and destroy them by the unique process of "membrane phagocytosis." This process, which is also described by many others including Policard and Bessis (1953), Weed and Reed (1966), and Croft *et al.* (1968), depends on the presence of anti-RBC antibodies which, following their union with erythrocytes, become cytophilic for macrophages and lead to the formation of rosettes. When macrophages and erythrocytes carrying such antibodies come in contact, the macrophages seemingly are able to pull off and phagocytize fragments of the red cells, leaving osmotically fragile erythrocytes which become spherocytic and undergo fragmentation. The antibodies in man known to be responsible for membrane phagocytosis are functionally incomplete IgG molecules. They do not fix C' or induce phagocytosis of whole erythrocytes, but after interaction with red cells they combine specifically with cytophilic receptors present on monocytes and mature macrophages, but not on granulocytes (Huber and Fudenberg, 1968).

In the mouse, a similar fragmentation of antibody-sensitized erythrocytes adhering to macrophages has been described (Lay and Nussenzweig, 1968). Results of this study indicate that macrophages of the mouse have surface receptors for complexes of antigen, xenogeneic antibody, and the first four components of C'. The combination of receptors on the macrophage with such complexes depended on the presence of divalent cations. Whereas, in this system, macrophage cytophilic receptors for 7S antibodies were resistant to trypsin treatment, the receptors for C' components were destroyed by trypsin. The existence of receptors on macrophage surfaces for antigen:antibody:C' complexes offers an additional mechanism for the efficient removal of sensitized erythrocytes and other materials from the body.

It is clearly evident that in autologous and allogeneic *in vivo* systems the nature of the antibody which sensitizes erythrocytes is of primary importance in determining the mode of the disposal of the erythrocytes. Of equal importance is the number of erythrocytes capable of being sensitized ("target" RBCs) as well as the relative number of RBCs present which do not bear the antigens specific for the antibodies used ("nontarget" RBCs). For example, if a small intravenous dose of Rh-positive RBCs coated with anti-D antibody is injected into a nonimmunized Rh-negative adult, membrane phagocytosis occurs and the cells are rapidly sequestered largely in the spleen (Jandl, Jones and Castle, 1957; Crome and Mollison, 1964). Since D antigenic determinants are sparse on the red cells, it is possible that the antibody coating of such cells is sufficient to permit their adherence to macrophages but is insufficient to permit phagocytosis. Stuart (1967) has proposed that the number of antibody molecules on the surface of erythrocytes may determine whether they merely adhere to phagocytes or are phagocytized. By contrast to the above experiment with incomplete IgG antibody, when a small number of Rh-positive RBCs is administered to an Rh-negative adult possessing complete IgM anti-D antibody, the RBCs are cleared less readily from the circulation and are sequestered primarily in the liver. Alternatively, in the ABO system where the antibodies are nonlytic complete agglutinins, if large numbers of incompatible cells are injected (as in a mismatched blood transfusion) the aggregates of agglutinated cells are removed from the circulation largely by macrophages of both the liver and lungs (Jandl, Jones, and Castle, 1957; Jandl and Tomlinson, 1958).

Thus, the nature of the antibodies and the degree of antibody-coating of RBCs are important in determining the site of the sequestration of RBCs (Jandl and Kaplan, 1960). Heavily coated RBCs tend to sequestrate in the liver, and lightly coated RBCs in the spleen.

4. Wound Healing

Macrophages are conspicuous in healing wounds and areas of tissue organization. They appear at the site of injury during the first few days, increase both in number and in maturity during following days, and decrease in number as fibrosis ensues. The emigration of blood monocytes into areas of organization, and their subsequent transition to mature macrophages, have been well documented by Ebert and Florey (1939). Other sources of the macrophages found in areas of healing are discussed in Chapter 4. Regardless of their source, macrophages function in the first stages of healing by invading the clot and by ingesting and digesting RBCs, fibrin, and cellular debris.

The sequence of cellular changes observed during wound healing illustrates the role of the macrophage in cell homeostasis, as discussed in Chapter 5. Granulocytes which first invade an injured area die and release cellular components which presumably facilitate the differentiation or the maturation of macrophages at the site. Ross (1964) found many extracellular granules, which appeared to be PMN granules, in wounds between the first and third day. He noted that macrophages were the predominating cell type in wounds at this time and that some of them contained bodies which appeared to be granules derived from PMNs. Macrophages also phagocytize whole dead PMNs. Substances are released from dying macrophages which stimulate fibroblast activity, resulting in fibrosis. During normal wound healing, fibrosis is minimal. However, in conditions in which excessive numbers of macrophages accumulate and die over a long period of time, fibrosis is excessive, e.g. in granulomatous diseases such as tuberculosis, sarcoidosis, silicosis, and histoplasmosis (Schowengerdt, Suyemoto, and Main, 1969).

B. *Regional Activities*

Macrophages in various regions of the body may have characteristic functions.

1. Peritoneum

The peritoneal cavity is normally sterile and the relatively small numbers of macrophages which can be collected from the healthy peritoneum appear to be relatively immature and inactive. Histological examination reveals depots of immature macrophages in milk spots of the omentum (Cappell, 1929b). During abnormal conditions, caused, for example, by bacterial infection or the introduction of particulates, large numbers of macrophages appear in the peritoneum. Many of these cells are mobilized from the omentum, others arise by division of existing macrophages (Aronson and Elberg, 1962), and still others may be derived from blood-borne immature precursors, as discussed in Chapter 4. Macrophages become highly activated following stimulation, i.e. they synthesize many lysosomes and frequently give evidence of extensive phagocytic activity. Extraneous material is rapidly cleared from the peritoneum by the phagocytic activities of macrophages and is usually digested intracellularly.

During the rejection of ascites tumor allografts (see Chapter 12) there is evidence that macrophages can kill tumor cells by a contact mechanism independent of phagocytosis, which results in the lysis of both macrophage and tumor cell. Later, other macrophages phagocytize and remove the cellular debris which remains (Baker *et al.,* 1962).

2. Lung

The environment in the lung differs greatly from that of the peritoneum. Not only is the milieu different, but also the stimuli encountered by alveolar macrophages are stronger and more numerous. Inhaled gases and particulates, including microbes, serve as strong stimuli to activate lung macrophages. Thus, it is not surprising that alveolar macrophages are normally more activated than peritoneal macrophages, even in germ-free animals (Leake and Heise, 1967). Although bacteria are not present in the germ-free environment, inhaled dusts and gases can serve as stimuli for macrophage activation.

Macrophages are vitally important in policing and clearing the lung of extraneous material. Green and Kass (1964) demonstrated that bacteria, labeled with P^{32} and given to mice in an aerosol, are quickly removed from the lung, largely by alveolar macrophages. Their data suggest that the action of the mucociliary stream serves to clear the lung of phagocytes containing ingested material. The ability of mice to clear bacteria from the respiratory tract is greatly inhibited by acute renal failure; Goldstein and Green (1966) postulated that this inhibition is caused by the biochemical changes known to occur subsequent to renal failure, which could adversely affect alveolar macrophage function. This might account for the observation that pulmonary infection is a frequent complication of renal failure.

A unifying hypothesis to explain the mechanisms of disposal of inhaled particles was presented by Heppleston (1963). From data obtained in experiments in which rats were exposed to hematite or silica dusts and examined at various time intervals, Heppleston drew the following conclusions. Nonmetabolizable particles, ingested by alveolar macrophages, are liberated upon death of the cell, and are rephagocytized by other alveolar macrophages. Movement of the alveolar fluid film toward sites of lymphatic drainage aids in the export of phagocytes containing ingested particles. After heavy exposure to dust, many particles remain in the alveoli for long periods of time. Dust foci enlarge and macrophage proliferation and disintegration continue; in the case of silica dust, fibrosis ensues. It is suggested that dusts enter the lymphatic system, either free or within macrophages, and localize in the hilar nodes.

Alveolar macrophages also contribute to immunity against viruses, by the production of interferon (see Chapter 6) and in other ways, discussed by Mims (1964a).

Increased numbers of macrophages, and a phenomenon known as "macrophage congregation" (Sherwin et al., 1968), are seen in lungs exposed to NO_2, an important component of polluted air. "Macrophage congregation" is defined as ". . . three or more 'spread' macrophages on a single epithelial cell." The extent of macrophage congregation was much greater in guinea pig alveolar cells exposed to 10 ppm NO_2 than in nonexposed cells. The significance of macrophage congregation is not clearly defined; however, it seems to reflect lung tissue damage. Cell selectivity was observed, in that some epithelial cells had many macrophages spread on their surfaces, while adjacent cells had none. Evidently damaged lung epithelial cells specifically attract alveolar macrophages, which congregate on their surfaces.

The observation that cigarette smoke depresses the *in vitro* antibacterial activity of rabbit alveolar macrophages (Green and Carolin, 1967) may be related to the effects of NO_2 or other gases in the cigarette smoke, since the active component of the smoke was soluble in water.

The lipid-containing alveolar macrophages studied by Bertalanffy (1964) differ in several ways from those without lipid inclusions. For example, their life span of 3 weeks within the lung is approximately three times that of nonlipid-containing alveolar macrophages, which are extruded from the lung within a week after mitosis. It was suggested that the lipid-containing macrophages remove cholesterol and other lipids from the blood while in intimate contact with lung capillaries, while alveolar macrophages without lipid inclusions function chiefly in the removal of particulate matter.

Macrophages throughout the body probably play a major role in maintaining the normal equilibrium of serum lipids (Bertalanffy, 1964; Day, 1967). There is also a remote possibility that alveolar macrophages may function in the production of lung surfactant, necessary for the integrity of this organ (see Chapter 6).

3. Central Nervous System

Normally the central nervous system (CNS) is not exposed to foreign material because the blood-brain barrier functions to effectively exclude the entrance of even many soluble substances into this system. When this barrier is breached, because of inflammation, trauma, or other causes, macrophages of the CNS soon become activated. As described in Chapter 2, microglial cells are the inactive stellate macrophages normally seen in the CNS. Following stimulation, they transform into typical ameboid, phagocytically active macrophages containing many lysosomes (Hosokawa and Mannen, 1963). These activated macrophages remove and digest materials in a manner analogous to that shown by peritoneal or alveolar macrophages.

Experimental allergic encephalomyelitis (EAE) can be produced in animals by injecting brain tissue or certain brain components incorporated in Freund's complete adjuvant. This disease resembles the human demyelinating disease, multiple sclerosis. Macrophages in the brain may contribute to the pathogenesis of EAE, as discussed in Chapter 12.

4. Lymphoid Tissue

Reticular cells of lymphoid tissue have been reported to have a nurse function for lymphocytes (see review by Trowell, 1965). It is postulated that lymphocytes with little cytoplasm and few mitochondria are so inactive that they have difficulty in generating enough energy to meet their requirements, and consequently must be supplied nutrients by nurse cells. Many investigators have observed contact and in some instances apparent continuity between lymphocytes and macrophages through cell processes. Trowell (1965) reviewed the evidence suggesting that macrophages transfer ATP or other cellular constituents to lymphocytes.

Macrophages in lymphoid tissue figure prominently in the removal of foreign material and its digestion into antigenic fragments (see Chapter 9). Macrophage-cytophilic antibodies are retained for long periods of time on dendritic reticular cells in lymph nodes, where they may promote the immune response by trapping and retaining antigen. Another interpretation of the observed spatial relations between lymphocytes and macrophages of lymphoid tissue is that RNA or RNA-antigen complexes are passed to lymphocytes by macrophages which have processed the antigen.

Tingible-body macrophages in lymph nodes and spleen also remove effete cells, such as plasma cells, which may be numerous during and following an active immunological response.

5. Testes

Carr, Clegg, and Meek (1968) summarized the literature on the Sertoli cell of the testes as a macrophage. Their electron micrographs clearly establish that Sertoli cells are typical macrophages, which remove extraneous materials and dead cells in seminiferous tubules. The possibility that they may function as nurse cells for spermatozoa is discussed by Trowell (1965).

6. Skin

Another type of macrophage postulated to have a nurse function is the melanophage of the skin (Trowell, 1965; Niebauer, 1968). Cells of this type apparently supply melanin to melanocytes in the skin.

7. Bone

Macrophages probably function in bone metabolism by serving as precursors of osteoclasts. Jee and Noland (1963) reported that charcoal, injected into the femurs of growing rabbits, was phagocytized by macrophages over the first 10 days. At 15 to 30 days a large number of charcoal-laden osteoclasts appeared, apparently formed by the fusion of macrophages. Jee and Nolan presented their data in support of the theory of Hancox (1949); namely, that phagocytic histiocytes can fuse to form osteoclasts. Data in conflict with this theory have been reported by Tonna (1963), and the question must remain open at present.

C. Additional Functions of Macrophages

1. Detoxification

Macrophages can detoxify certain substances. For example, highly toxic but slightly soluble granules of arsenic trisulfide, when administered intraperitoneally to laboratory animals, are taken up by macrophages and degraded into nontoxic compounds which are excreted in the urine. The same amount of arsenic trisulfide, however, is fatal to the recipients if it is placed in sacs within the peritoneum where it is protected from phagocytosis and detoxification by macrophages but instead can be released in a soluble toxic form (Metchnikoff, 1905).

The powerful exotoxin of diphtheria kills cultured spleen, kidney, or peritoneal macrophages from nonimmunized guinea pigs within 24 hours (Frolova and Sokolova, 1964). In contrast, peritoneal and splenic macrophages from immune animals are highly resistant to the toxin and remain viable and mobile in its presence. Attempts were made to determine whether cytophilic antibodies could account for these results. Nonimmune guinea pig macrophages were exposed to horse serum diphtheria antitoxin, washed, and tested with dilutions of toxin. Since no protection was afforded by this procedure, it was concluded that cytophilic antibodies do not contribute to the observed immunity against diphtheria toxin. However, the cells were from guinea pigs and the serum antibodies were of horse origin, hence it is possible that cytophilic antibodies were present but not demonstrable because the cytophilic receptors of guinea pigs and horses differ. It would be of interest to reinvestigate this question in the light of recent advances in the understanding of cytophilic antibody activity (see Chapter 10).

Rutenburg, Schweinburg, and Fine (1960) determined that macrophages can detoxify endotoxins from *E. coli in vitro*. Ravin *et al.* (1960) showed that bacterial endotoxins are absorbed from the intestinal tract of normal rabbits and of rabbits in the state of hemorrhagic shock. Such absorbed endotoxins remain in the serum of shocked animals. Schweinburg and Fine (1960) demonstrated that fatal endotoxemia develops because the RES is unable to destroy absorbed endotoxins during conditions of shock induced in several ways. Wiznitzer *et al.* (1960) reported that the normal RES removes and rapidly inactivates circulating endotoxin; however, the RES damaged by blockade or by reversible hemorrhagic shock can remove only a small amount of circulating toxin and is able to detoxify very little of the removed material. In addition, there is evidence that the development of tolerance to the toxic effects of endotoxins depends on enhanced activity of the RES (Freedman, 1960).

Ballantyne (1967) postulated that esterase activity of RES cells may contribute to the detoxification of endotoxins and of potentially toxic lipids produced during metabolism associated with extensive cellular mitosis. Macrophages may also indirectly influence the detoxification of barbiturates (DiCarlo *et al.,* 1965; Barnes and Wooles, 1968).

It has been postulated that iron in macrophages plays a role in the detoxifying activities of these cells. Janoff (1964) suggested that iron may act in two ways, first to activate lysosomal enzymes and second to neutralize toxins. The acid pH and accumulation of reducing substances within phagolysosomes would favor release of iron for both of these functions.

2. Inactivation of Thromboplastin

Blood thromboplastin prepared *in vitro* and administered to an intact animal of the sames species (rat) is cleared from the circulation by the RES (Spaet *et al.,* 1961). It has also been reported that rabbit peritoneal macrophages can inactivate rabbit blood thromboplastin in an *in vitro* system, while alveolar macrophages have no effect (Arakawa and Spaet, 1963). It was concluded that the laboratory-prepared thromboplastin used was treated as foreign particulate material by the RES. No evidence was presented concerning similar activity under normal physiological conditions.

The RES has been implicated in the *in vivo* production of a hypercoagulable state in dogs (Rabiner and Friedman, 1968). This state is defined as an increased tendency of the blood to clot intravascularly because of alteration of its constituents. This alteration can be created experimentally by infusing autologous hemolyzed RBCs (hemolysate). Depression of RES function by pretreatment with carbon or by splenectomy accentuated the hypercoagulable state. It was postulated that the augmentative effect of RES depression on the state of hypercoagulability induced with hemolysate could be related to lack of clearance of liberated coagulant particles.

SUMMARY: Macrophages, frequently aided by the activity of opsonins, act as scavengers to dispose of foreign and effete cells and other materials. They can degrade and reutilize many of the ingested substances, thereby contributing to the conservation of stores of iron, turnover of serum proteins, nutrition of cells, and resorption of tissue. Wound healing depends, in part, on the scavenger activities of macrophages; in addition, macrophages may influence the homeostasis of fibroblasts and thus indirectly affect the healing process and fibrosis.

Within the peritoneum, macrophages are normally inactive but can be stimulated to proliferate and to become highly activated. Such macrophages readily clear the peritoneum of extraneous material. Alveolar macrophages are normally more activated than peritoneal macrophages and function in clearing the lung of inhaled particles, producing interferon, and other activities. Macrophages in other locations throughout the body may have specialized functions unique to their location.

Other functions of macrophages include: detoxification of certain simple chemicals, exotoxins, and endotoxins; possibly the regulation of clotting under certain special conditions; and immunological activities (discussed in other chapters).

Chapter 9

The Role of Macrophages in the Antibody Response

The importance of macrophages in the antibody response has been recognized for virtually as long as the response has been studied. Although originally it was postulated that macrophages might be the site of antibody synthesis (see review by McMaster, 1953), present evidence indicates that they do not produce antibodies (Storb and Weiser, 1968). However, they contribute to the antibody response in several important ways. Macrophages trap, process, and store antigens. In addition, they can present specific information to antibody-forming cells in the form of a fragment of antigen coupled to ribonucleic acid (RNA), or possibly in other ways. These functions have been studied extensively, both *in vivo* and *in vitro*.

A. Contributions of Macrophages to the Antibody Response in Vivo

Both the initiation and extent of the antibody response are influenced greatly by the route of entrance of the antigen into the body and its subsequent fate. The fate of antigen varies depending on numerous factors, including its dose and solubility, and previous exposure of the host to the antigen.

The fate of radioactively labeled bovine gamma globulin (BGG) injected i.v. into rabbits has been traced by Dixon *et al.* (1953) and serves as a classical example of the disposition of a soluble antigen. The injected BGG initially equilibrates between vascular and extravascular fluids and is not concentrated or retained in appreciable amounts by any tissue; nevertheless, enough is taken up to stimulate antibody production. By approximately the fourth day, when specific antibodies appear, the labeled BGG rapidly complexes with antibody and is eliminated from the circulation, so that by about day 7 the antigen is cleared completely and free serum antibodies are demonstrable. If the antigen is again introduced while circulating antibodies are still present, it is cleared within 1 to 2 days. Even though antibodies may no longer be measurable in previously sensitized animals, reintroduction of the antigen results in an anamnestic response, and antigen is cleared in an accelerated manner within 4 days. When antigen and antibody combine, the complexes are rapidly removed and catabolized by phagocytic cells of the RES.

Particulate antigens are cleared from the circulation by cells of the RES, as described in Chapter 7. Their fate depends on a number of factors, such as the size of the particles and the presence of either natural or immune antibodies.

Following their primary injection, some antigens are retained over long periods within cells of the RES, but others are catabolized quickly and are no longer demonstrable within cells (Dixon *et al.,* 1953; Ehrenreich and Cohn, 1968a).

1. Antigen Trapping

Nossal, Ada, and Austin (1964a, b) have used the flagella of certain *Salmonella* species and their soluble subunits, flagellin, as antigens. Since both are easily labeled and highly antigenic, they are ideally suited for studies on the fate of either particulate or soluble antigen. Nossal, Ada, and Austin (1964b) demonstrated that particulate flagella are first trapped by macrophages which line the medullary sinuses of lymph nodes draining the injection site. Soon thereafter, antigen appears in primary lymphoid follicles in the cortex of the nodes. By combining electron microscopy with radioautography, Ada *et al.* (1967) showed that a primary dose of flagella is taken up by typical macrophages of the lymph node medulla. Within the cell, antigen, either free or in pinosomes, becomes surrounded by tiny lysosomal vesicles and is completely enclosed within lysosomal structures by 30 minutes after injection. These lysosomes fuse to give rise to large pinolysosomes which persist in the medullary macrophages for 6 weeks or longer. Although PMNs are present in the nodes they do not participate to an appreciable extent in antigen uptake. In cortex of the lymph nodes, trapped antigen is adsorbed to fine dendritic processes of reticular cells, which appear to be nonphagocytic macrophages; here it may be retained for as long as 2 weeks following its primary administration. This association allows close contact between lymphoid cells and antigen on the surface of macrophages.

Ada *et al.* (1967) described a third type of cell, the tingible-body macrophage, which is capable of trapping flagellar antigens, especially during the secondary response. This cell retains label within myelin inclusions.

When soluble flagellin is used instead of intact flagella, the antigen is seen throughout the node soon after its primary subcutaneous introduction. One to 2 days later, it becomes localized in a manner similar to that observed with flagella within an hour after injection (Ada *et al.,* 1967).

The fate of soluble antigen bearing a radioactive label has been followed by Szakal and Hanna (1968), using electron microscopic radioautography. Szakal and Hanna noted that the antigen became localized on highly convoluted infoldings of splenic reticular cells (macrophages) in lymphoid follicles during the primary response in the mouse spleen. Villous extensions of ribosome-rich "immunoblasts" were observed in close association with antigen on macrophage surfaces. Demonstrable antigen decreased from 20 to 30 days after administration, and by 30 days was no longer detectable.

The localization of antigen within lymphoid follicles has been observed by many other investigators (see review by McDevitt, 1968). This pattern of antigen trapping appears to result from the reaction of antigen with cytophilic antibodies on the surfaces of dendritic macrophages. The amount of antigen captured increases as antibody is formed; passively transferred antibodies also cause a marked follicular localization of antigen (Lang and Ada, 1967). There is also evidence that the Fc portion of the IgG antibody molecule is largely responsible for the reaction of IgG with the macrophage membrane, as would be expected for cytophilic antibodies (Ada *et al.,* 1967).

2. Antigen Processing

As described above, macrophages ingest and sequester soluble antigen within pinolysosomes. Particles such as SRBCs, a complex of different antigens, are also ingested and processed by macrophages. The question of whether macrophage intervention contributes or is necessary to antibody formation has been approached experimentally. It is, of course, possible that macrophages which degrade erythrocytes, bacteria, or other particulate antigens are simply fulfilling their role as scavengers and play no part in antibody formation. That this is not the case has been demonstrated by many studies which have shown that inhibition of RES function reduces the extent of the antibody response, and, conversely, that stimulation of RES function leads to increased antibody production (e.g. Thorbecke and Benacerraf, 1962; Stuart and Davidson, 1964; Franzl and McMaster, 1968a, b). Thus, it is well established that macrophage activity facilitates antibody production by retaining and processing antigen, as well as in other possible ways.

The processing of a bacterial antigen, streptococcal M protein, by macrophages was studied by Gill and Cole (1965). It was postulated that particles containing a complex of antigens are phagocytized and processed into small antigenic moieties. Other streptococcal antigens, the group-specific polysaccharide of Group A, may also be processed by macrophages; an enzyme for the hydrolysis of this substance has been described in rabbit alveolar macrophages (Ayoub and McCarty, 1968).

The ability of macrophages to process antigen for antibody production may not be expressed in newborn animals. Braun and Lasky (1967) reported that intraperitoneal (i.p.) injection of adult peritoneal macrophages and antigen (SRBCs) into 2-day old syngeneic mice results in an antibody response, whereas SRBCs alone do not induce antibody production in mice until 5 to 10 days after birth. Similar results were reported by Argyris (1968), who concluded that the immunological immaturity of newborn mice may result from lack of antigen recognition or processing by macrophages, rather than from lack of immunocompetent cells.

The experiments of Frei, Benacerraf, and Thorbecke (1965) provided evidence that macrophage processing of antigen is an important step in the induction of the antibody response, at least to certain antigens. These investigators demonstrated that serum, containing soluble antigen left in the circulation after RES clearance of phagocytizable antigen particles, could be transferred to other animals to produce tolerance or an impaired immune response. The usual extent of antibody formation was restored by administering heat-denatured antigen, which is avidly phagocytized. These results indicated that macrophage processing of antigen is essential for the induction of the normal extent of antibody formation.

Other evidence suggesting that macrophage activity is essential in some, but not all, types of immune responses was reviewed by Mitchison (1969). The experimental results reported by Mitchison led to the conclusion that certain protein antigens are more potent in stimulating a primary antibody response when processed by macrophages than when free.

Feldman and Gallily (1967) found that macrophages are indispensable in the primary response against *Shigella* antigens. Purified populations of mouse peritoneal macrophages, incubated *in vitro* with *Shigella* organisms, induced antibody formation when transferred to sublethally x-irradiated recipients. In lethally x-irradiated mice, passive transfer of normal lymphocytes, plus macrophages that had been primed with *Shigella,* induced antibody formation; however, neither type of cell was effective alone. Following x-irradiation, macrophages were fully capable of phagocytosis, but appeared to lack the capacity to so process antigen that it could signal antibody production. Thus, macrophage processing is essential to the primary immune response in this system. The work of Pribnow and Silverman (1967) supports the conclusion that macrophage processing of antigen is necessary for stimulating antibody synthesis.

Conflicting results have been obtained in other systems, indicating that the nature of the antigen, and perhaps other factors, may determine whether macrophage activity is essential for the induction of antibody synthesis. In experiments similar to those discussed above, it was found that reconstitution of the immune response to SRBCs could not be accomplished by transferring normal macrophages, incubated with SRBCs, to sublethally irradiated recipients; reconstitution of the response to *Shigella* was, however, achieved with normal macrophages incubated with *Shigella* antigens (Gershon and Feldman, 1968). Although Askonas and Rhodes

(1965) found that the immunogenicity of hemocyanin was increased when it was complexed with macrophage RNA, they did not determine whether macrophage processing is essential for the primary antibody response to this antigen.

Unanue (1968) used anti-macrophage serum to remove macrophages from a mixed cell preparation, and reported that the lymphocytes which remained were able to make antibodies to hemocyanin. This suggested that macrophages are not essential for the antibody response to this large antigen molecule. These reports emphasize the difference in responses obtained using various antigens and different experimental systems.

Anti-macrophage serum (AMS) may prove to be a valuable tool for studying the activities of the macrophage in antibody production and other functions. The AMS prepared by Unanue (1968) was specific for macrophages and did not react with lymphocytes or erythrocytes. Others have reported studies with AMS (Panijel and Cayeux, 1968; Jennings and Hughes, 1969; Loewi et al., 1969; Heise and Weiser, 1969); the antiserum is not always specific for macrophages but may also react with lymphocytes or erythrocytes to some extent.

Animals made tolerant to an antigen during neonatal life have macrophages which can take up the antigen and process it. When such antigen-containing macrophages are transferred from the tolerant animal to a normal host, antibody production to the specific antigen is stimulated (Harris, 1967). This indicates that macrophage capabilities need not be abrogated during the tolerant state. On the other hand, the genetic capacity to respond to antigen with antibody formation may be expressed in macrophage activities. Mice genetically incapable of responding to certain synthetic polypeptide antigens can form specific antibodies if they are given RNA extracted from peritoneal exudate cells of responder animals which have been incubated with the antigen (Pinchuck et al., 1968). The activity of the RNA was RNAase-sensitive, and the RNA contained small amounts of antigen which were not sufficient to elicit antibody formation alone. These experiments demonstrate that tolerance can occur at the macrophage level; they also indicate the necessity of macrophage processing of this antigen.

Overall, it would appear that macrophage processing is essential for the initiation of the primary antibody response to some antigens, but not to others. No definite conclusions can be drawn concerning the physical or chemical properties of the antigen which determine whether it will require processing by macrophages.

The manner of transfer of processed antigen to immunocompetent cells is not clearly defined. Continuity between macrophages and lymphocytes has been described (e.g. Aronson, 1963; Schoenberg et al., 1964) and could account for the passage of information-containing material between cells. However, there is no reason to believe that direct passage of information is required for antibody production. Some other possible modes of transfer of processed antigen or information are discussed in the review by Sulitzeanu (1968).

Antigen may be presented to potential antibody-forming cells by dendritic macrophages which have trapped the antigen. The presence of macrophage-cytophilic antibodies greatly facilitates such a mechanism, especially during the secondary response.

The intracellular fate of antigen may depend on the state of activation of the macrophage which engulfs it. For example, Cohn (1964) observed that the antigenicity of *E. coli* was destroyed more readily by highly activated BCG-induced alveolar macrophages than by less activated oil-induced peritoneal macrophages of rabbits. Blanden (1968) reviewed evidence provided by several investigators suggesting that antigen ingested by hyperactive macrophages may become so completely degraded that it is no longer antigenic, and immunodepression results. Immune macrophages can be activated by antigen; it is possible that such activation serves as a homeostatic mechanism and contributes to control of antibody synthesis.

3. Antigen Storage

In experimental animals, antigen is retained in detectable amounts over periods of time which vary greatly with the nature of the antigen. For example, Sabin (1939) found that azoprotein was sequestered within macrophages but only remained visible for a few days after antibodies became manifest. Felton (1949) demonstrated that pneumococcal polysaccharides can persist in tissue for years, perhaps throughout the lifetime of the animal. Garvey and Campbell (1957) showed that protein antigens persist in tissue for months, perhaps bound to RNA. Using the sensitive test of reverse anaphylaxis, McMaster and Kruse (1951) were able to detect soluble antigens in tissues for months after their administration. They found that, following its intravenous injection, antigen was stored within widely distributed cells of the RES.

Peritoneal macrophages of mice take up labeled hemocyanin (MSH), and degrade 90% of it within 2 to 5 hours (Unanue and Askonas, 1968). The remaining MSH is retained within the macrophages in an immunogenic form for at least 2 weeks.

Many experiments have been performed to ascertain the fate of antigen and its retention in animals that form antibodies and in those that fail to form antibodies. Campbell and Garvey (1963) reviewed the literature on this subject, including much of their own work. More recently, Ada *et al.* (1967) demonstrated that labeled antigen remains in medullary macrophages and associated with dendritic reticular cell membranes in lymph nodes for at least several weeks. They postulated that this represents a mechanism for trapping and conserving antigen within lymphoid follicles, and may serve to generate memory cells within the nodes over extended periods.

4. Influence on Cellular Homeostasis

It has been reported that macrophage lysates can stimulate the proliferation of plasma cells (see Chapter 5, Section C). The various interrelations between macrophages and other cell types, although not clearly understood, suggest that the macrophage or its products exert a profound influence on the homeostasis of the cell types involved in antibody production.

B. Contributions of Macrophages to Antibody Production in Vitro

For many years attempts were made to initiate antibody production by isolated cells *in vitro*. Although Carrel and Ingebrigtsen (1912) reported that antibodies can be produced in culture by bone marrow and lymph node cells, the attempts of others to repeat their experiments gave varied results. In 1948, Fagraeus demonstrated beyond doubt that antibodies can be produced *in vitro*. She showed that explanted spleen fragments, rich in plasma cells, mount a typical secondary antibody response. Many other investigators subsequently reported antibody synthesis in organ and cell cultures derived from animals previously given antigen (see review by Dutton, 1967).

1. Studies with Whole Cells

In vitro, the initiation of a primary response is much more difficult to attain than the stimulation of secondary antibody production. Stevens and McKenna (1958), Globerson and Auerbach (1965), Tao and Uhr (1966), Mishell and Dutton (1966), and Mosier (1967) are among those who have demonstrated antibody production by normal lymphoid cells in culture. In every instance the cultures contained more than one type of cell.

The necessity of the participation of two cell types in the *in vitro* initiation of the antibody response was emphasized by Mosier (1967), who separated mouse spleen cells into apparently macrophage-rich and lymphocyte-rich populations, on the basis of adherence or nonadherence to the culture vessels, and showed that only mixed populations of cells responded to a primary exposure to SRBCs. Thus, at least with particulate antigens as complex as SRBCs, macrophage processing may be essential for the initiation of antibody synthesis. However, the possibility exists that the adhering cells are not all macrophages. In similar experiments Mosier (1969) was unable to identify the cells morphologically.

Moore and Schoenberg (1968) also presented evidence suggesting that macrophage activity is required for initiation of a primary, but not a secondary, antibody response. Nine months after primary immunization of rabbits with horse spleen ferritin when no formation or persistence of antibody could be detected, lymph node cells were collected and used for *in vitro* studies. Relatively purified suspensions of lymphocytes, separated from macrophages by passage through a glass-bead column, could respond to secondary stimulation with antigen by synthesizing specific antibody. Thus, although macrophages were necessary to initiate a primary response *in vitro* in this system, they were not required for the secondary response. In fact, their presence appeared to inhibit the secondary response, presumably because they degraded antigen which might otherwise have stimulated the primed lymphocytes directly.

2. Studies with Subcellular Components

The role of macrophage RNA in the immune response was discussed in a review by Fishman and Adler (1967). The work of Fishman (1959, 1961) and Fishman and Adler (1963) suggested that antibody formation requires the interaction of two types of cells. It was proposed that antigen is processed by macrophages and that information-containing RNA is transferred to potential antibody-forming cells. Phenol extracts, made from peritoneal exudate cells which had been incubated with antigen, initiated a primary antibody response by cultured lymphoid cells. The activity was RNAase sensitive, suggesting that the RNA of macrophages plays a crucial role in antibody production. The active material could have been messenger RNA (mRNA) or RNA complexed with antigen, the complex serving as a "super-antigen." Askonas and Rhodes (1965), using radioactively labeled hemocyanin as antigen, demonstrated that RNA extracts prepared from mouse peritoneal macrophages which had ingested the hemocyanin contained antigen or antigen fragments; nevertheless the activity of the extracts was RNAase sensitive. They found that, although most of the antigen taken up by macrophages is rapidly degraded, a small amount is demonstrable within these cells for many days. It was suggested that RNA binds a fragment of antigen and enhances its uptake by potential antibody-forming cells, or alternatively protects it against digestion by lysosomal enzymes.

Similar results have been obtained by Cohen and Parks (1964), Friedman (1964), Chiller (personal communication) and Abramoff and Brien (1968), using SRBCs as antigen, immunogenic RNA from mixed cell populations, and the Jerne plaque assay for antibody-forming cells. Gottlieb, Glišin, and Doty (1967), Abramoff and Brien (1968), and Chiller, observed that activity of immunogenic RNA extracts was destroyed by either RNAase, pronase (devoid of RNAase activity), or specific antibody, suggesting that antigen fragments in the complex lend specificity and that RNA serves some other unknown but essential function.

The results of hybridization of macrophage DNA with RNA from macrophages which had ingested antigen, reviewed by Gottlieb (1968), do not favor the existence of a unique mRNA. Furthermore, immunologically active RNA may be less than 5S (M.W. < 24,000), whereas the RNA needed to code for only the light chain of an antibody molecule would have to be of a molecular weight (M.W.) of 180,000 or higher. Another reason to doubt that macrophage RNA, as described above, acts as a specific messenger for antibody production is that macrophages have not been shown to synthesize antibodies and therefore would not be expected to produce mRNA coding for antibody molecules.

Recent evidence of Adler, Fishman, and Dray (1966) is in accord with the possibility that RNA from peritoneal exudate cells may serve as specific messenger for a fragment of antibody light chain bearing an allotypic marker. Gottlieb (1968) distinguished the properties of this RNA from those of the macrophage-RNA discussed above, and concluded that this RNA may be specific mRNA derived from lymphocytes, rather than macrophages, in the peritoneal cell population studied.

On the basis of the evidence available at present it is concluded that:

1. In no case has RNA from macrophages been definitely established as messenger RNA for specific antibody formation.

2. RNA which can act as messenger for the production of specific antibody molecules or for portions of antibody molecules bearing a given allotypic marker probably has been derived from lymphocytes, rather than macrophages, in the mixed populations of cells used.

3. RNA could protect antigenic fragments and allow their persistence within macrophages over long periods of time.

4. RNA, complexed with antigen, could aid in the entrance of antigen into, or its presentation to, immunologically competent cells, thus endowing the complex with the property of a "super-antigen" able to cause enhanced antibody production.

SUMMARY: Macrophages contribute to the antibody response in several ways. They trap antigen in draining lymph nodes, either by pinocytosis or phagocytosis, or both, and by retention of antigen on their membranes. Macrophages may process antigen into more highly antigenic fragments or complexes, and they can store antigen in some form for long periods of time.

In vitro, the primary antibody response to certain antigens depends on the interaction of at least two cell types, apparently macrophages and lymphocytes. Macrophages may be essential for the primary response to complex antigens; at least they enhance the primary response. However, the secondary response is not enhanced by macrophage activity, and may even be depressed. Extracts of RNA from antigen-containing cells, predominately macrophages, can serve as "super-antigens" to induce an enhanced primary antibody response. It remains to be determined whether the active RNA is derived from the large proportion of macrophages or the small proportion of lymphocytes in the preparations.

Chapter 10

Antibodies Cytophilic for Macrophages

NOT UNTIL the present decade has the importance of cytophilic antibodies been realized. Boyden and Sorkin (1960, 1961) introduced the term "cytophilic," which is used to designate affinity for cells. They described cytophilic antibodies, formed by rabbits in response to human serum albumin, which in the free state had an affinity for certain cells in a mixed population of cells from the spleens of normal rabbits. The sites on antibodies responsible for their affinity for cells are independent of the sites which bind antigen. The characteristics of several kinds of antibodies which exhibit cytophilia for various kinds of cells are outlined in a general consideration of cytophilic antibodies presented by Weiser, Myrvik, and Pearsall (1969). The present discussion will be limited to antibodies that are cytophilic for macrophages, including both naturally occurring antibodies and antibodies resulting from known antigen stimulation.

The teleological necessity for a mechanism of discriminating between indigenous and foreign material by animals was discussed by Boyden (1962). Clearly, it is essential that phagocytes which dispose of foreign or effete autologous material must have a recognition mechanism for distinguishing between these materials and viable cells of self. Boyden (1960) postulated that humoral recognition factors (antibodies) could fulfill this role, either by coating the particle to be phagocytized or by first attaching to the phagocyte. Subsequently it was demonstrated that humoral antibodies of certain classes can be adsorbed by the membranes of macrophages before combining specifically with antigen. Thus macrophages can bear on their surfaces specific recognition factors in the form of cytophilic antibodies which promote the adherence and phagocytosis of antigen-bearing particles. As North (1968) has speculated, the macrophage may need to recognize only the cytophilic attachment sites of antibody molecules in order to recognize and phagocytize any type of particle. Rowley (1962) reviewed the evidence which suggests that opsonins are always required for effective phagocytosis by macrophages; Benacerraf (1968) has postulated that under proper circumstances all cytophilic antibodies may act as opsonins to promote phagocytosis.

Boyden (1964) produced antibodies cytophilic for macrophages, by administering sheep red blood cells (SRBCs) in Freund's complete adjuvant to guinea pigs. The resulting antibodies combined with receptors on macrophages and were then able to bind SRBCs to give the appearance of rosettes. Boyden (1963) summarized much of the earlier literature on this subject.

There is no evidence to prove that macrophages synthesize the antibodies found on their surfaces, although this has not been definitely ruled out. Instead, it is probable that cytophilic antibodies are synthesized by lymphoid cells and are transferred to macrophage membranes via serum and possibly by some other unknown mechanism involving cell contact. It is known that some classes of humoral antibodies are specifically cytophilic for macrophages (see Section B of this chapter), so that at present there is no necessity to invoke other possible mechanisms to account for the acquisition of such antibodies by macrophages. However, Sharp and Burwell (1960) reported that marked peripolesis, i.e. "wandering of lymphocytes around macrophages," occurred in cultures of cells from lymph nodes draining a skin homograft, and in spleen cell cultures several days after the i.v. administration of antigen. Because peripolesis was never noted in cultures derived from normal nonstimulated lymphoid tissue, it is probably related to immunological events. The attraction involved in peripolesis is unexplained, but the process represents a mechanism for intimate contact between lymphoid cells and macrophages. It is conceivable that extensive transfer of cytophilic antibodies from lymphocytes to macrophages could occur during cell contact. Such a mechanism would greatly facilitate the arming of macrophages with cytophilic antibody. The results of Holub and Hauser (1969), suggesting that alveolar macrophages produce antibodies could be explained in part by such a mechanism.

Macrophage cytophilic antibodies vary in certain of their characteristics, depending on factors such as the species of origin and the route and schedule of antigen administration. Moreover, within a species macrophage cytophilic receptors for IgG and IgM antibodies may differ. There is also variation in the receptors on macrophages of different animal species.

A. Characteristics of Antibodies Cytophilic for Macrophages

The literature on macrophage cytophilic antibodies has been reviewed by Nelson and Boyden (1967) and Nelson (1969). Guinea pig, rabbit, and mouse cytophilic antibodies were characterized by Berken and Benacerraf (1966), who demonstrated that most if not all of the $7S\gamma_2C'$-binding antibodies of guinea pigs were cytophilic for guinea pig macrophages. The formation of cytophilic antibodies was favored by the use of Freund's complete adjuvant and these antibodies could be eluted from macrophages by incubation at 37° C for 45 minutes.

Both 7S and 19S fractions of rabbit and mouse antisera have been tested for cytophilia for macrophages of the corresponding species and in each instance only 7S antibodies reported to be cytophilic (Berken and Benacerraf, 1968). The observation that pepsin digestion completely destroys the cytophilic properties of $7S\gamma_2$ antibodies demonstrated that the macrophage-binding site is on the Fc segment of the molecule (Berken and Benacerraf, 1966).

Nelson and Mildenhall (1968) studied the production of guinea pig macrophage cytophilic antibodies induced by varied schedules of antigen administration. They used SRBCs in Freund's complete adjuvant, a combination known to elicit delayed hypersensitivity in guinea pigs. When the antigen emulsion was administered intraperitoneally, intradermally, or into the foot pads, high titers of macrophage cytophilic antibodies were obtained at 2 weeks and the animals exhibited pronounced delayed reactions to antigens given intradermally. Subcutaneous injection of the antigen-adjuvant emulsion resulted in negligible titers of cytophilic antibody and mild delayed skin sensitivity to antigen at 2 weeks. In a series of experiments there was, in general, a lack of correlation between the extent of the delayed skin reaction and the titer of demonstrable cytophilic antibody in the serum at the time of testing. Nelson and Mildenhall have also found that macrophage cytophilic antibodies are largely in the $7S\gamma_2$ globulin fraction of guinea pig serum. Their conclusion that cytophilic antibodies are not important in delayed sensitivity reactions will be discussed in the following chapter.

Gowland (1968) presented evidence that, although most of the guinea pig cytophilic antibodies to SRBCs are present in the $7S\gamma_2$ globulin fraction of serum, not all $7S\gamma_2$ antibodies are cytophilic.

Mouse cytophilic antibodies may differ in some respects from those of the guinea pig. Nelson, Kossard, and Cox (1967) reported the existence of two kinds of cytophilic activity in mouse antisera. Whereas "early antibody" was present in serum collected 7 days after a single primary dose of antigen and was present when delayed sensitivity was demonstrable, "late antibody" was present in hyperimmune serum collected after secondary immunization and was not associated with the presence of delayed sensitivity. The early cytophilic antibody is apparently not a conventional immunoglobulin, but late cytophilic antibody in hyperimmune serum is a $7S\gamma_2$ immunoglobulin, as in the guinea pig. Cytophilic antibodies of mice, active in immunity against *Salmonella typhimurium,* are mercaptoethanol-sensitive and appear to be IgM (Rowley, Turner, and Jenkin, 1964).

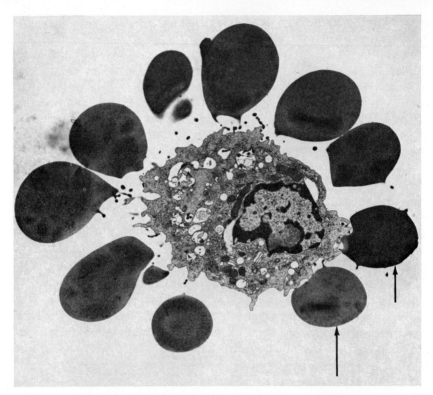

FIGURE 10-1. Rosette formation caused by the reaction of red cell antigen with cytophilic antibodies on the surface of a macrophage. Electron micrograph of a macrophage collected from the lymph node of a guinea pig immunized with sheep red blood cells (SRBCs) in Freund's complete adjuvant 5 days before the micrograph was taken. The macrophage has been allowed to react *in vitro* with the antigen (SRBCs), and a section has been cut through the resulting rosette. The arrows indicate SRBCs that are adherent to the macrophage in this section; the space between the other SRBCs and the macrophage results from a sectioning artifact. All 10 SRBCs in the photograph are adhering to the surface of the macrophage. The bits of red cells present in clear spaces within the macrophage probably do not represent phagocytized material, but rather are the result of sectioning. Magnification: 6,000. (Courtesy of U. Storb and V. Chambers.)

These findings suggest that immunoglobulins of various classes may be cytophilic for macrophages. Furthermore, the properties of the cytophilic antibodies of each class may differ. In general, $7S\gamma_2$ globulin antibodies which are cytophilic for macrophages appear to act as opsonins to facilitate phagocytosis; in addition they may have other functions. The mouse, but not the guinea pig, has cytophilic antibodies which are not conventional immunoglobulins and which appear to be correlated with the presence of delayed sensitivity.

B. *Nature of Macrophage Receptors and the Cytophilic-Binding Reaction*

Macrophage receptors for cytophilic antibodies show both intraspecies and interspecies differences. Mouse hyperimmune sera contain antibodies which are cytophilic for both mouse and guinea pig macrophages; however, guinea pig cytophilic antibodies are not cytophilic for mouse cells, suggesting that at least two kinds of antibody receptors are present on guinea pig macrophages. Other inhibition data likewise suggest that macrophages may possess a variety of receptors both for allogeneic and xenogeneic antibodies (Kossard and Nelson, 1968a). In this regard, it should be emphasized that the actions of antibodies across species barriers have no necessary significance with respect to natural events within the species.

Enzyme treatment has been used to remove cytophilic antibody from macrophages and expose receptors on the cells. Mild trypsin treatment presumably removes and destroys adherent cytophilic antibody, because, following trypsinization, attraction for specific antigen is lost and the cell is capable of adsorbing antibodies of other specificities (Han, 1966; Heise, Han, and Weiser, 1968). In accord with this presumption, trypsinization increases the ability of normal macrophages to adsorb specific cytophilic antibodies, evidently by removing existing bound antibody molecules and freeing the cytophilic receptors (Howard and Benecerraf, 1966; Han, 1966).

It has been reported that natural and early cytophilic antibodies are easily removed from macrophages by trypsinization but that late cytophilic antibodies are resistant to removal (Nelson and Cox, unpublished data quoted by Nelson and Boyden, 1967).

With respect to the susceptibility of macrophage cytophilic receptors to enzymes, Kossard and Nelson (1968b) have found that papain treatment of normal guinea pig macrophage monolayers has little effect on the susceptibility of such monolayers to sensitization by guinea pig cytophilic antibodies. Neither did papain treatment alter the capacity of sensitized macrophages to combine with the specific antigen, SRBCs. Similarly, mouse macrophages treated with papain or with trypsin were able to absorb at least as much "late" hyperimmune cytophilic antibody from serum as nontreated macrophages. Mouse "early antibodies" in serum collected 7 days after immunization reacted in a markedly different manner. They were cytophilic for untreated macrophages but not for enzyme-treated macrophages. This suggested that mouse macrophages have different types of receptors. Some of the receptors, specific for early cytophilic antibodies, are sensitive to trypsin and papain, and other receptors, specific for late cytophilic antibodies, are resistant to these proteolytic enzymes.

Other important studies on the nature of peritoneal macrophage receptors for cytophilic antibodies have been conducted by Davey and Asherson (1967). These investigators injected a single dose of SRBCs in Freund's complete adjuvant into the footpads of guinea pigs and collected sera 3 weeks later. Macrophage receptors for the cytophilic antibodies produced in this manner were destroyed by phospholipase A and by chemical treatments which alter lecithin. Treatment of macrophages with proteolytic enzymes, such as pronase, ficin, trypsin, and chymotrypsin, caused increased adherence of cytophilic antibodies to the treated macrophages, while neuraminidase and lipase had little effect. It was concluded that, in the guinea pig, phospholipid or phospholipoprotein is an important component of macrophage receptors for cytophilic antibodies.

Evidence suggesting that human monocytes possess specific receptors for IgG antibodies complexed with erythrocytes has been presented by LoBuglio, Cotran, and Jandl (1967), Huber and Fudenberg (1968), and Cline and Lehrer (1968).

The affinity of cytophilic antibodies for macrophage receptors is relatively weak, compared with the affinity of these antibodies for antigen. Cytophilic antibodies vary markedly in their avidity for the macrophage surface; it has been shown that many of them are readily eluted from cell surfaces only at temperatures above 37° C, e.g. 56° C for 30 minutes (Boyden and Sorkin, 1961; Granger and Weiser, 1966; Heise, Han, and Weiser, 1968). In other instances, cells may rapidly lose their cytophilic antibody by elution during incubation at 37° C unless serum containing cytophilic antibody is present in the medium (Berken and Benacerraf, 1966; Nelson and Boyden, 1967; Kossard and Nelson, 1968a).

The union of guinea pig macrophage receptors with cytophilic antibodies is poor at 4° C and is favored by increases in temperature in the range from 4° C to 37° C. Variation in pH from 5.7 to 8.1, or addition of a chelating agent, has no effect on association of cytophilic antibodies with macrophages (Berken and Benacerraf, 1968).

Upon its reaction with antigen, cytophilic antibody shows a striking increase in affinity for the macrophage (Berken and Benacerraf, 1966). It is postulated that this enhanced affinity may be due to allosteric changes in the antibody molecule which favor its cytophilic binding, or to a stabilization of binding to the macrophage brought about by the simultaneous reaction of several molecules of antibody with adjacent antigenic determinants. Indeed it is possible that antibody with little or no cytophilia when in the free state may become markedly cytophilic when combined with antigen. The term "cytophilic antibodies," by definition, should not be used to describe these antigen-antibody complexes, but should be reserved to denote antibodies which in the free state are cytophilic. It has also been shown that C' complexed with antigen and antibody can contribute to the cytophilia of antigen-antibody complexes in certain circumstances (Uhr, 1965; Huber *et al.,* 1968).

It is probable that many cytophilic antibodies, with specificities for a variety of antigens, exist in normal serum and compete for macrophage receptor sites. Experimental evidence supporting this hypothesis has come from studies which show that nonimmune sera can inhibit the adherence of specific cytophilic antibodies present in an immune serum (Berken and Benacerraf, 1968; Cline and Lehrer, 1968). Kossard and Nelson (1968a) speculated that, in the *in vivo* environment, macrophage membranes are saturated with cytophilic antibodies in equilibrium with those in the serum. Consequently, in the case of macrophages from immune animals, a substantial proportion of the cytophilic antibodies on the surfaces of these macrophages would be expected to be specific for the antigen used for immunization. "Desensitization of macrophages" (i.e. loss of specific cytophilic antibodies) by incubation at $37°$ C in nonimmune serum was postulated to result from an equilibration between cytophilic antibodies of other specificities present in the serum and the specific immune antibodies bound to the macrophage. An alternative possibility is that the serum in the medium may stimulate pinocytosis and thus speed the turnover of cell membrane, with consequent desensitization resulting from endocytosis of preexisting cytophilic antibodies. Current evidence suggests that a combination of these events occurs in macrophage desensitization.

C. Significance of Antibodies Cytophilic for Macrophages

Antibodies cytophilic for macrophages may play a role in antibody production by contributing to antigen trapping. Natural cytophilic antibodies to SRBCs have been found in the sera of some normal guinea pigs (Nelson and Boyden, 1967); such natural antibodies could aid in trapping antigen during the primary response. It is clearly evident that immune cytophilic antibodies are important in capturing antigen during the secondary response (Ada *et al.,* 1967).

Although some investigators disclaim that cytophilic antibodies contribute significantly or play a causal role in delayed sensitivity reactions, others hold the opposite view. The question has not been answered definitively and will be considered in more detail in the next chapter. Since macrophage cytophilic antibodies are diverse in character it is possible that conflicting opinions reflect, in part at least, differences in the varieties of antibodies under study.

It is reasonably certain that $7S\gamma_2$ cytophilic antibodies formed late after the administration of antigen are concerned with opsonization and phagocytosis (Parish, 1965; Benacerraf, 1968). The value of such a mechanism for carrying antibodies into areas of infection where humoral antibodies may not readily penetrate is obvious. Since the competition between cytophilic antibodies in the serum for sites on macrophages involves cytophilic antibodies of all specificities, macrophages which reach an area of local antibody formation should become rapidly and preferentially coated with specific cytophilic antibody or with complexes of antigen and antibody. Hence, from the standpoint of cellular immunity, macrophages bearing cytophilic antibodies probably represent an important mechanism of defense.

SUMMARY: The biological and physicochemical properties of macrophage cytophilic antibodies from animals of several species are discussed. Receptors for cytophilic antibodies on guinea pig macrophages are composed of phospholipids, perhaps in combination with other compounds. The affinity of cytophilic antibodies for macrophage receptors is relatively weak, compared with their affinity for antigen. The reaction of antigen with cytophilic antibody enhances the cytophilic affinity of the antibody for macrophage receptors, probably because of allosteric changes in the antibody molecule and other possible reasons.

Cytophilic antibodies of different specificities in the serum are in dynamic equilibrium with antibodies bound to receptor sites on macrophages. Antibodies cytophilic for macrophages contribute substantially to phagocytic defense mechanisms and probably to cellular immunity as well.

Chapter 11

The Macrophage in Delayed Sensitivity *

MACROPHAGES are important in the induction of states of delayed sensitivity and in delayed sensitivity reactions. The reviews by Benacerraf (1965), Uhr (1966), Humphrey (1967), Spector (1967), and Turk (1967) provide an excellent survey of the literature on delayed sensitivity; therefore, only a brief discussion of the subject will be included here for the benefit of those unfamiliar with the field. Major emphasis will be placed on the contributions of macrophages to delayed sensitivity.

The term "delayed sensitivity" is used to designate a type of sensitivity characterized by reactions which are delayed in onset following administration of the test reagent. These reactions involve an inflammatory response in which mononuclear cells predominate. Delayed sensitivity can be passively transferred with cells but not with serum. The prototype is the cutaneous tuberculin reaction elicited by a purified protein derivative (PPD) of old tuberculin. When an animal sensitized with tubercle bacilli is injected intradermally with PPD, a skin reaction characterized by erythema and induration becomes apparent in 6 to 12 hours and reaches a peak at 24 to 48 hours. Histological examination of the test site shows that, although mononuclear cells and PMNs infiltrate concurrently, PMNs predominate early in the response before the skin lesion becomes visible. This early PMN response is transient and is followed by a predominance of mononuclear cells, including many proliferating macrophages (Spector, 1967). Turk, Heather, and Diengdoh (1966) observed that macrophages account for more than half of the infiltrating mononuclear cells at 24 hours, whereas by 48 hours 70% are lymphocytes.

One hypothesis put forward to explain the delay in the cutaneous tuberculin reaction is that the delay represents the time necessary for infiltrating sensitive cells to accumulate at the test site. This possibility is ruled out by the observation that the systemic tuberculin reaction, in which the

---

* The term "delayed sensitivity" is used in preference to the more commonly used term "delayed hypersensitivity."

antigen is injected intravenously or intraperitoneally, is likewise delayed. In this instance tuberculin should rapidly reach sensitive cells everywhere. It is more likely that the delay in both local and systemic reactions represents the time needed for recruitment and activation of normal cells by antigen-triggered sensitive cells, and for subsequent events. It is known that nonsensitive cells are recruited to participate in delayed reactions because animals depleted of lymphocytes, by x-irradiation or other means, do not accept passive transfer of delayed sensitivity. Moreover, passive transfer experiments with labeled cells from sensitive animals have shown that very few of the cells which accumulate at the cutaneous site are transferred cells.

In addition to tuberculin, other substances known to elicit delayed sensitivity reactions include many other microbial antigens (such as histoplasmin, coccidioidin, and brucellergen), other extraneous antigens (such as primrose, poison ivy, and simple chemicals), and the antigens of allografted tissues. Sensitivities which arise as the result of contact of the sensitizing substance with an integument, e.g. a simple chemical in contact with the skin, are called "contact sensitivities."

Present evidence indicates that there is a close, and possibly a causal, relation between delayed sensitivity and allograft immunity, and between delayed sensitivity and autoimmune diseases. That such a relationship exists between delayed sensitivity and antimicrobial cellular immunity is much less certain.

One of the major distinguishing characteristics of delayed-type sensitivities, mentioned above, is that these sensitivities can be transferred with cells but not with serum. By contrast, sensitivities involving humoral antibodies can usually be transferred with serum. Although humoral antibodies are not known to contribute to delayed sensitivity reactions, it would appear that some type of antibody activity is involved because of the specificity of the reactions and because agents known to suppress antibody formation also suppress the development of delayed sensitivity. For these reasons, the concept of a role for cell-bound antibody (cell-associated antibody) in delayed sensitivity reactions has evolved. Such antibody may never leave the cell which produces it and could belong to a special immunoglobulin class. Alternatively, it could be a strongly cytophilic antibody which might be passed to macrophages by cell contact.

Three unique features of delayed sensitivities are that they can be induced by proteins but not by polysaccharides, that cellular antigens most readily induce sensitivity when whole cells are used rather than portions of cells, and that the reaction sites of antigen and hypothetical antibody are large—in the case of hapten-carrier complexes they encompass not only the hapten but a contiguous portion of the protein carrier as well.

There can be no doubt that lymphocytes are intimately involved in the initiation of delayed sensitivity. Recent evidence also strongly supports the concept that macrophages contribute to reactions of delayed sensitivity. Turk (1967), Dumonde (1967a), and Dumonde, Howson, and Wolstencroft (1968) have reviewed the literature on the role of the macrophage in delayed sensitivity.

A. Studies in Vivo

In common with the classical antibody response, the delayed sensitivity response can be separated into three components. The first is the phase concerned with the afferent limb of the response, during which antigen is transported to the draining lymph nodes and other sites of antibody formation. The second is the central response, which is concerned with antibody synthesis and activation of effector cells. The third, or efferent limb, of the response comprises the interaction of effector cells with target antigen.

There is little doubt that the macrophage functions in the afferent limb of the delayed sensitivity response, both by transporting antigen and by processing it. If it can be assumed that the allograft reaction represents a delayed sensitivity reaction (Brent, 1958; Billingham and Silvers, 1963; Turk, 1967) it may then be used as a model of delayed sensitivity. It has been shown (Barker and Billingham, 1968) that lymphatic communication from skin allografts to draining lymph nodes is essential for sensitization, presumably because this is the principal avenue by which graft antigens reach the sites of the central immune response. The development of contact sensitivity also demands that lymphatic connections between the skin exposed to antigen and the draining lymph nodes must be intact (Landsteiner and Chase, 1939; Frey and Wenk, 1957). Macrophages probably contribute by transporting, trapping, and processing antigen in draining lymph nodes. Depression of the activity of macrophages by large doses of trypan blue results in a modest prolongation of graft survival time (Brent and Medawar, 1961), as does pretreatment of graft recipients with silica to destroy macrophages (Pearsall and Weiser, 1968a). Such treatments interfere with the afferent limb of the response.

It is well known that certain adjuvants, such as the mycobacteria in Freund's complete adjuvant mixture, exert a strong "directive effect" in channeling the response to protein antigens incorporated in the mixture toward delayed sensitivity (Dienes, 1932). Wilkinson and White (1966) discussed this phenomenon and reported their observations on a similar directive effect produced by bentonite. Mycobacteria, bentonite, and certain other adjuvants produce three events which appear to be related, i.e. the development of macrophage-epithelioid granulomas, increased γ-2 globulin production, and delayed sensitivity to the protein accompanying the adjuvant. Reid and Mackay (1967a) have also emphasized the association between granulomatous inflammation and the development of delayed sensitivity. This association suggests that the macrophages of the granuloma contribute in some way to the development of delayed sensitivity and γ-2 globulin production. The possibility that γ-2 globulin functions as a cytophilic antibody in delayed sensitivity reactions has been disputed.

Granuloma formation depends on the physical state of the inducing agents, especially their particulate state, as well as upon their biochemical properties (Reid and Mackay, 1967b). Within granulomas, epithelioid cell formation is induced by foreign materials which the macrophage has difficulty in digesting, such as peptidoglycolipids of mycobacteria (Pernis, Bairati, and Milanisi, 1966). It has been suggested that epithelioid cells have a high degree of induced digestive capacity and capability for processing antigens.

The mechanisms by which macrophages contribute to the development of delayed sensitivity are unknown but could be related to antigen processing or to some special manner of presenting processed antigen to the inducible cell. Burnet (1968) has postulated that in order to initiate the state of delayed sensitivity it may be necessary for antigen to be presented to the inducible cell by membrane contact with a mobile "inducer" cell carrying the antigen on its surface. The macrophage is well-fitted to function as an inducer cell because of its capacities to process antigen and to carry adsorbed antigen on its surface.

In contrast to the directive effect of adjuvants favoring the induction of delayed sensitivity is "immune deviation," a state in which certain humoral antibodies are formed but delayed sensitivity does not develop (cf. review by Asherson, 1967). Immune deviation is produced by injecting alum-precipitated antigen, or antigen in saline, prior to the administration of adjuvant-antigen mixture. Suppression of γ-2 antibody production often occurs concomitant with suppression of the delayed sensitivity response; however, these two events are not invariably linked, thus disfavoring the possibility that γ-2 antibody is essential for the expression of delayed sensitivity (Borel, Fauconnet, and Miescher, 1967). Immune deviation could involve feedback mechanisms of homeostasis, regulating the development of delayed type sensitivity. In this situation it is not unreasonable to expect that antibodies of one class may exert control over the production of other classes of antibody, as is the case with suppression of IgM antibody production by IgG antibodies. However, to date passive transfer of immune deviation with serum has not been achieved (Asherson, 1967). Tuberculous guinea pigs, which give no indication of immune deviation, are deficient in anaphylactic sensitivity to tuberculoproteins, hence it is possible that anaphylactic (IgE-like) antibodies could be responsible for immune deviation. However, the most likely possibilities are that immune deviation results either from a deviation of antigen away from cells which would respond to produce delayed sensitivity, or from a direct effect of antigen in blocking the response of such cells. The finding that lymphoid cells from animals in a state of immune deviation have a reduced capacity to passively transfer delayed sensitivity (Borel, Fauconnet, and Miescher, 1967) indicates that these cells are directly affected.

The central response to antigen concerned with the development of delayed sensitivity probably occurs principally within the draining lymph nodes. Turk (1967) reviewed the changes which occur in lymph nodes during the development of delayed sensitivity. In the corticomedullary (thymus-dependent) areas, large pyroninophilic cells (LPCs) develop in response to antigen. These cells have high metabolic activity; they synthesize both DNA and RNA and divide to give rise to small lymphocytes similar in appearance to the precursors of LPCs. Sensitized cells leave the lymph nodes by way of the efferent lymphatics (Hall and Morris, 1965) and reach the blood stream.

The efferent limb of the delayed sensitivity response is undoubtedly mediated by sensitized cells from the lymph nodes which reach the site of antigen deposition (e.g. tuberculin in the skin, or the transplanted graft); however, the precise mechanisms by which the delayed sensitivity reaction is effected remain a mystery. It is known that many lymphocytes, LPCs, and macrophages congregate at the reaction site, and that macrophages proliferate there (Spector, 1967). It is also well established that peritoneal exudate cells or preparations of circulating leukocytes containing lymphocytes can passively transfer delayed sensitivity (Landsteiner and Chase, 1942; Humphrey, 1967). It is the consensus that passive transfer can be achieved with lymphocytes alone; indeed Dumonde, Howson, and Wolstencroft (1968) have passively transferred delayed sensitivity with lymphocyte suspensions containing less than 1% macrophages.

The exact function of the large number of macrophages and lymphocytes in reaction sites is not clear. One possibility is that sensitized lymphocytes migrate from lymph nodes via the circulation to the test site and act as the principal effector cells responsible for the reaction; macrophages may then contribute to the reaction in some secondary manner or function merely as scavenger cells to remove the products of tissue damage. It is known that, when sensitized lymphocytes are cultured with specific antigen, blast transformation occurs and a nonspecific factor(s) is liberated (see Section B of this chapter). This factor causes inhibition of macrophage migration *in vitro* and is nonspecifically cytotoxic; it also produces inflammatory reactions similar to delayed-type sensitivity reactions when injected into guinea pig skin (Bloom and Bennett, 1968; Chandler, Heise, and Weiser, 1969). If lymphocytes at the local test site form cytotoxin, the cytotoxin could contribute to the delayed reaction, either by its inflammatory effects or by its effects on macrophages, e.g. attracting them to the area, immobilizing them, and inducing their proliferation. In fact it has been reported that a factor chemotactic for macrophages is liberated from sensitive lymphocytes stimulated with antigen (Ward and David, 1969), and it is known that macrophages are immobilized and proliferate at reaction sites (Dumonde, 1967b).

Another possibility is that macrophages possess cytophilic antibody and effector activity at the time they arrive at the test site (see review by Nelson and Boyden, 1967). *In vivo* observations which are compatible with this concept have come from the investigations of Nelson and co-workers (Nelson and Boyden, 1963; Nelson and North, 1965; Nelson, 1965), who described a "macrophage disappearance reaction" characterized by the disappearance of macrophages from the peritoneal fluid of sensitive animals within a few hours after administration of antigen. This disappearance of macrophages from the peritoneal fluid is caused by clumping of the macrophages to each other and by adherence of the clumps to serosal surfaces. The specificity of the reaction suggests that it may result from the binding together of macrophages bearing cytophilic antibody.

Holtzer and Winkler (1967) and Holtzer (1967) produced a state of delayed sensitivity to SRBCs in guinea pigs, without accompanying serum cytophilic antibodies. Some animals gave delayed skin reactions to an extract of SRBCs when they had no demonstrable serum hemolysins and no cytophilic antibodies, either in serum or on cells; conversely, reactions to skin tests were often negative when the serum contained cytophilic antibodies. It was concluded that delayed sensitivity is unrelated to the occurrence of cytophilic antibodies. Since, in these tests for the presence of cytophilic antibodies on macrophages, the cells were allowed to spread on glass for 1 hour before exposing them to SRBCs, it is possible that cytophilic antibodies were lost from the cells by elution and by membrane endocytosis.

Reports of successful transfer of tuberculin sensitivity with highly purified preparations of alveolar macrophages from sensitized animals also suggest that macrophages can act as effector cells in delayed sensitivity reactions. In a few experiments, Han (1966) apparently succeeded in transferring a limited degree of delayed sensitivity to tuberculin with macrophages. He used a cell suspension derived from BCG-sensitized albino guinea pigs (consisting of 95 to 98% macrophages and 1 to 2% lymphocytes), containing the equivalent of 1 ml of packed alveolar macrophages, injected intracardially. The recipients were skin tested immediately with 10 μg of PPD and gave weak but typical delayed tuberculin reactions. Control animals given 20 times as many lymphocytes of splenic origin as were found to contaminate the macrophage preparations failed to respond with a positive reaction to the skin test. Despite these results with control preparations, it is possible that lymphocytes present in the suspensions of sensitive macrophages contributed to the transfer and that macrophage preparations devoid of lymphocytes would not passively transfer delayed sensitivity.

In the experiments described above, it was necessary to inject the macrophages into the left side of the heart, presumably to prevent the rapid sequestration of cells in the lung or other organs. Studies on the fate of intravenously injected macrophages derived from the mouse peritoneum (Roser, 1965), lung (Russell and Roser, 1966), and liver (Roser, 1968) have indicated that many of the transferred cells localize in the liver of recipients.

Heise and Weiser (unpublished results) used a local method for transferring tuberculin sensitivity. They found that positive skin reactions result when 10^7 cells from BCG-sensitized guinea pigs, either alveolar macrophages, lymph node lymphocytes, or peripheral leukocytes, were mixed with 10 μg of PPD and administered intracutaneously. Both donors and recipients in these experiments were inbred strain-13 guinea pigs, and the macrophage preparations were approximately 95% pure. Lymphocytes were separated from the suspensions of alveolar cells; it was found that control animals, given a dose of lymphocytes equivalent to the number contaminating the macrophage preparation used, failed to develop a reaction. In all of these passive transfer experiments it is possible that lymphocytes acted synergistically with macrophages and that if pure macrophage suspensions devoid of all lymphocytes could be prepared they would not be effective.

Attempts by others to transfer delayed sensitivity with purified macrophage preparations have usually failed. An occasional positive result has been obtained in strain-2 guinea pigs; however, some investigators have alleged that the local reactions reported resemble Arthus reactions more than delayed sensitivity reactions (Turk, 1967).

Peritoneal exudates are rich in thymus-dependent lymphocytes derived from the circulation. Lymphocytes from the peritoneum can be 10 to 20 times as effective as lymph node lymphocytes in transferring delayed sensitivity (Dumonde, Howson, and Wolstencroft, 1968). Hence, among peritoneal exudate cells, which are highly effective in passive transfer of delayed sensitivity, it is probable that the lymphocyte is the principal effector cell.

Thus, the results of *in vivo* studies strongly support the concept that macrophages are important in the afferent limb of the delayed sensitivity response, probably by virtue of transporting and processing antigen and presenting it to the immunocompetent cells responsible for delayed sensitivity. Macrophages may also contribute, in a minor way at least, to the efferent limb of the delayed sensitivity response because of cytophilic antibodies on their surfaces, or possibly for other reasons. Presumably any effector role of macrophages possessing cytophilic antibodies would be the result of antibodies with the strongest cytophilic affinity.

B. *Studies in Vitro*

Currently, several tests are being used to study delayed sensitivity reactions *in vitro,* and each of them involves macrophage activity to some extent. Unfortunateiy, none of these tests has been shown to correlate well with the degree of delayed sensitivity as measured by the standard skin test. The best studied of the *in vitro* tests is the macrophage migration-inhibition test; another in wide use is the lymphocyte blast-transformation reaction. Mitosis of immune macrophages following exposure to antigen is also an *in vitro* phenomenon ascribed to delayed sensitivity, and may provide a basis for determining delayed sensitivity.

The literature on the inhibition of migration of macrophages has been reviewed by Turk (1967) and David (1968a, b). Many years ago it was observed that the migration of cells from tissue explants of sensitized animals was inhibited during exposure to antigen. This observation formed the basis for the development of a capillary tube method for the semi-quantitative determination of inhibition of migration of mixed populations of cells, e.g. peritoneal exudate cells (George and Vaughan, 1962; David *et al.,* 1964a). Suspensions of washed cells are placed in capillary tubes and the tubes are sealed at one end; the tubes are centrifuged gently to sediment the cells and are then broken at the interface between cells and supernatant fluid. The cells within the tubes are cultured in small Mackaness chambers for 24 to 48 hours. In the presence of antigen, normal macrophages migrate to form a monolayer on the glass around the open end of the tube. However, in the presence of antigen, sensitized macrophages are inhibited in their migration from the tubes. The extent of inhibition of migration is taken as a rough measure of the degree of sensitivity of the cells. David *et al.* (1964a, c) postulated that the test measures delayed sensitivity for several reasons. First, there is usually a correlation between migration-inhibition reactions and specific delayed skin reactions. Second, the migration-inhibition reaction is antigen specific and, in the case of a hapten bound to a carrier, exhibits specificity for the carrier-hapten complex. Moreover the methods of immunization used to produce sensitized cells also produce delayed sensitivity, as measured by the skin test. Conversely, methods of immunization which lead to the production of high titers of circulating antibody do not cause delayed sensitivity, as measured by skin tests or by migration-inhibition tests. David and co-workers concluded that migration inhibition represents a delayed sensitivity reaction *in vitro* and that cytophilic antibodies do not play an important part in the reaction (David, 1968a, b).

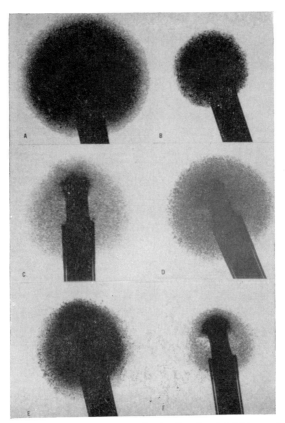

FIGURE 11-1. The role of cytophilic antibody in the inhibition of migration of purified macrophages by specific antigen. Purified alveolar macrophages from tuberculin-sensitive guinea pigs were "disarmed" by removal of cytophilic antibodies with trypsin and "rearmed" by exposure to heat-eluted antibodies from sensitive macrophages. The cultures in the right-hand column were exposed to 20 μg PPD per milliliter. *A* and *B* represent sensitive control macrophages. *C* and *D* represent "disarmed macrophages." *E* and *F* represent "rearmed macrophages." (Courtesy of E. R. Heise.) (From Weiser, Myrvik, and Pearsall: "Fundamentals of Immunology." Lea & Febiger, Philadelphia, 1969.)

Similar conclusions were reached by Thor (1968) and Thor and Dray (1968a) who reported that a positive correlation exists between delayed sensitivity skin reactions in man and migration inhibition reactions obtained with lymph node cells.

It is not necessary for all of the cells in a population to be sensitive in order to obtain migration inhibition. David and co-workers (1964b, d) obtained positive migration-inhibition tests when as few as 2.5% sensitive cells were mixed with a population of nonsensitive cells. They also showed that trypsinization of sensitive cells temporarily abolishes their sensitivity to the migration-inhibition test.

Thor and Dray (1968b) reported that normal human lymph node cells can be sensitized to the migration-inhibition test with an RNA extract of human lymph node cells from tuberculin-sensitive donors. The active factor in the extract was between 4S and 28S, was RNAase-sensitive, and contained a small amount of protein. Although the concept that the active factor is RNA was favored, the possibility that it is a fragment of antigen coupled with RNA was not ruled out.

The cause(s) of migration inhibition remains an open question. David (1966, 1968a,b) and Bloom and Bennett (1966, 1968) characterized a soluble migration inhibitory factor (MIF) which is produced by culturing sensitized lymphocytes for from 6 hours to 2 days in the presence of antigen. The synthesis of MIF can be interrupted by adding puromycin to the culture medium. Only the lymphocytes from animals displaying delayed sensitivity produce MIF. The factor is capable of causing inhibition of migration of normal macrophages; it is nondialyzable, trypsin-sensitive, stable to heating at 56° C for 30 minutes, and it has a molecular weight of ca. 70,000. It was postulated that, in migration-inhibition reactions produced with mixed-cell populations, two cell types interact to produce the inhibition; i.e. sensitized lymphocytes, on exposure to antigen, produce MIF, which in turn inhibits the migration of macrophages.

The conclusion that macrophage migration inhibition is a reliable indicator of delayed sensitivity has been challenged. Amos et al. (1967) reported that cytophilic antibodies from serum can passively sensitize normal macrophages to the migration-inhibition test. Their results were confirmed by Heise and Weiser (1969). Amos and co-workers suggested that not all of the mechanisms involved in migration inhibition are associated with delayed sensitivity, and emphasized that it is not safe to assume that the test measures only the degree of delayed sensitivity.

Studies by Dumonde et al. (1968), designed to elucidate the relative roles of lymphocytes and macrophages in delayed sensitivity reactions, indicate that sensitive lymphocytes are the primary effector cells in such reactions and that macrophages are "innocent bystanders." These investigators observed that the capacity of a cell mixture to passively transfer delayed sensitivity *in vivo,* as well as to confer sensitivity on normal populations of cells *in vitro,* was correlated with the relative number of lymphocytes, but not macrophages, present in the mixture. However, it is possible that the method they used to purify cells on glass-bead columns may have abrogated to some extent the capacity of macrophages to participate in reactions of delayed sensitivity (see Chapter 10). They postulated that sensitized lymphocytes bear specific receptors which react with antigen, and in consequence release, not only substances which promote lymphocyte mitosis, but also a macrophage-immobilizing factor(s), which functions *in vivo* to arrest macrophages at the site of antigen deposition. It is also possible that the local release of chemotactic substances and macro-phage-cytophilic antibodies by antigen-triggered lymphocytes augments the contribution of macrophages to the cutaneous reaction.

Other investigations on the role of MIF in the migration-inhibition reaction and the cutaneous tuberculin reaction have been carried out by Heise and Weiser (unpublished results), using alveolar cells from tuberculin-sensitive inbred guinea pigs. Heise and Weiser's findings are essentially in agreement with those of David discussed above and, in addition, indicate that MIF is probably identical with the cytoxin produced by lymphocytes, described by Granger and Williams (1968). The MIF does not kill macro-phages under conditions which result in migration inhibition (Bloom and Bennett, 1968). Preliminary experiments have indicated that cytotoxin in high concentration kills syngeneic macrophages, but in lower concentrations causes activation of the macrophages, as indicated by increased size and numbers of lysosomes which stain for acid phosphatase (Pearsall and Weiser, unpublished results).

Weiser and associates (1969) demonstrated that two mechanisms can contribute to the inhibition of migration of macrophages in the tuberculin system, namely MIF and the reaction of antigen with cytophilic antibody on the surface of sensitive macrophages. When cytophilic antibodies on sensitive macrophages in a purified preparation were removed by trypsin treatment, the cells were no longer sensitive to the migration inhibition test; susceptibility could be restored by exposing the trypsinized macro-phages to immune serum or to cytophilic antibodies eluted from sensitized macrophages by heating at 56° C for 30 minutes. Normal macrophages could also be passively sensitized to the migration-inhibition test, especially if they were first trypsinized.

The observation of Fauve and Dekaris (1968) that the spreading of tuberculin-sensitive macrophages on glass can be inhibited by tuberculin probably depends on mechanisms similar to those involved in macrophage migration inhibition.

A second *in vitro* phenomenon purported to be a good indicator of delayed sensitivity is the blast transformation of sensitive lymphocytes which occurs following exposure of the lymphocytes to antigen (see review by Oppenheim, 1968). Some data indicate that certain antigens must be processed by macrophages before they can cause lymphocyte transformation (Hersh and Harris, 1968; Gordon, 1968). There are several reasons for concluding that blast transformation reflects delayed sensitivity. One of these is the observation that the specificity of lymphocyte blast transformation with antigen parallels that of other delayed sensitivity reactions. Furthermore, in the course of sensitization, lymphocyte blast transformation can be demonstrated before a positive skin reaction can be elicited, suggesting that it is the more sensitive indicator of delayed sensitivity.

Other evidence does not favor the conclusion that lymphocyte blast transformation measures only delayed sensitivity (see review by Turk, 1967). Antigen-stimulated blast transformation can be induced in lymphocytes from animals with either immediate or delayed sensitivity. In addition, blast transformation occurs in response to phytohemagglutinin and various other substances, presumably by mechanisms independent of antigen stimulation. These observations make it difficult to conceive of the procedure as being a dependable measure of delayed sensitivity, even though it may often accurately reflect such sensitivity (Turk, 1967).

A third possible *in vitro* indicator of delayed sensitivity is the increased mitosis of sensitized macrophages following exposure to specific antigen. Forbes and Mackaness (1963), and others, have reported that sensitive macrophages ordinarily have a very low mitosis rate *in vitro,* but when stimulated by antigen they exhibit increased mitosis. This indicates that macrophages are specifically involved in delayed sensitivity reactions, and suggests the possibility that the increased mitosis rate among sensitive macrophages exposed to specific antigen might be a useful indicator for measuring delayed sensitivity.

Certain observations made earlier by other investigators may be related to the phenomenon of antigen-stimulated mitosis of macrophages. Waksman and Matoltsy (1958) showed that the addition of antigen to cultures of peritoneal cells from sensitized guinea pigs produces a marked increase in the number of macrophages present after 24 hours, as compared with control cultures without antigen. This was ascribed in part to better survival of sensitive cells in the presence of antigen, and in part to the maturation of mononuclear cells and the limited proliferation of macrophages. An early decrease in total cell count at 18 to 24 hours was caused by the disappearance of large mature macrophages; the subsequent increase in macrophages was attributed to the maturation of intermediate-size mononuclear cells into typical macrophages. It was suggested that similar events *in vivo* could account for the proliferation of macrophages noted to occur around small veins during delayed sensitivity reactions. These favorable effects of antigen on sensitive peritoneal cells in culture did not correlate regularly with the results of migration-inhibition tests with spleen cells from the same animals. Whether antigen exerts a favorable or a cytotoxic effect on sensitive cells appears to depend largely on certain experimental conditions, such as antigen dosage and type of medium employed.

Svejcar and Johanovsky (1961a, b, c) confirmed the above *in vitro* observation that the addition of appropriate amounts of specific antigen to cultures of sensitive peritoneal cells accelerates the maturation of macrophages and prolongs their survival.

In antigen-containing cultures of mixed populations of cells, consisting of many macrophages and relatively few lymphocytes, it is possible that several events take place. The sensitive lymphocytes present probably respond to antigen with blast transformation and the production of cytotoxin. Cytotoxin may kill some macrophages, resulting in a decrease in cell number. However, simultaneous antigen stimulation of the sensitized macrophages probably induces mitosis, so that by 24 hours the total number of cells in the culture begins to increase. Thus the increased number and greater survival of sensitized peritoneal macrophages in the presence of antigen could be a reflection of proliferation and subsequent maturation of macrophages over an extended period of time.

At present, it is not possible to relate these *in vitro* activities of lymphocytes and macrophages directly to events in delayed sensitivity reactions *in vivo*. The question of whether macrophages of sensitized animals can act *in vivo* as effector cells, independent of lymphocytes, remains unanswered. However, it has been shown beyond reasonable doubt that macrophages function as specifically immune cells, both *in vivo* and *in vitro*, in immune reactions in which delayed sensitivity is thought to be of paramount importance (such as allograft rejection).

In light of this evidence, obtained from experiments both *in vitro* and *in vivo*, it may be postulated that the following sequence of events occurs in the prototype of delayed sensitivity reactions, the cutaneous tuberculin reaction. Injection of tuberculin into the skin of a sensitized animal results in a migration of both sensitive and nonsensitive cells into the test site. Among the sensitive cells are lymphocytes which respond to antigen with blast transformation, the production of MIF (cytotoxin), and possibly the production of other contributing substances, including cytophilic antibody. Some of these substances are chemotactic for PMNs and macrophages, attracting many of them into the area. Depending on the concentration, lymphocyte cytotoxin could induce inflammation, kill cells at the test site, and immobilize and activate macrophages. Inasmuch as normal animals depleted of lymphocytes cannot accept passive transfer of tuberculin sensitivity, some substances provided by antigen-triggered sensitive lymphocytes must induce normal lymphocytes to contribute to the reaction. Presumably the contribution of normal lymphocytes is an active one and is not limited to mere infiltration of the test site. Cytophilic antibody on macrophages arriving at the test site, or provided to them locally by lymphocytes, could contribute by reacting with antigen to cause macrophage proliferation. This complex of responses could account for the two major components of the reaction, namely inflammation and induration.

SUMMARY: Macrophages probably function in the induction of delayed sensitivity by trapping, transporting, and processing antigen. In addition they may present information to inducible cells in some special way, such as by contact of their antigen-carrying membranes with the membranes of the inducible cell. Macrophages may contribute as effector cells to delayed sensitivity reactions, by virtue of adsorbed cytophilic antibody.

States of delayed sensitivity have been passively transferred with suspensions of relatively pure (95 to 98%) macrophages. Despite the purity of the preparations, transfer may have depended on the activity of the lymphocytes which inevitably contaminate macrophage preparations, or on synergism between macrophages and lymphocytes in the preparation, rather than the activities of macrophages alone.

In vitro tests which commonly reflect states of delayed sensitivity include the inhibition of migration of macrophages, the inhibition of macrophage spreading, lymphocyte blast transformation, and the mitosis of sensitive macrophages.

Chapter 12

Macrophages and Acquired Cellular Immunity*

THE TERM "acquired cellular immunity," usually referred to simply as "cellular immunity," is used in this monograph to define that immunity which results from the effector activities of cells rather than from humoral antibodies, and which can be transferred with cells but not with serum.

The two principal types of cellular immunity, anti-tissue and antimicrobial, have certain characteristics in common. For example, both depend on the effector activities of immune cells and both are commonly engendered only or most effectively with living cells rather than dead cells or cell components. Despite these common characteristics, a clear distinction

---

* The terminology currently used to describe different types of tissue transplantation is presented in the table below. The old terms are given along with the preferred new terminology:

Terminology Used in Tissue Grafting

Old Noun	Old Adjective	New Noun	New Adjective	Definition
autograft	autologous	none	none	Recipient receives graft of his own tissue
isograft	isologous	syngraft	syngeneic	Recipient receives graft from a genetically identical or near identical donor of the same species (identical twin or inbred animal)
homograft	homologous	allograft	allogeneic	Recipient receives graft from a genetically dissimilar donor of the same species
heterograft	heterologous	xenograft	xenogeneic	Recipient receives graft from a donor of another species

From Weiser, R. S., Myrvik, Q. N., and Pearsall, N. N.: "Fundamentals of Immunology for Students of Medicine and Related Sciences." Lea & Febiger, Philadelphia, 1969.

should be made between anti-tissue and antimicrobial cellular immunity. Whereas antimicrobial cellular immunity depends on the activities of macrophages as effector cells against intracellular parasites, anti-tissue cellular immunity depends on the effector activities of both lymphocytes and macrophages.

The states of delayed sensitivity and cellular immunity usually develop concomitantly, which suggests that they may be causally related and that delayed sensitivity may be an essential component of cellular immunity. Although this concept has been disproved in the case of antimicrobial cellular immunity, it may be true of anti-tissue cellular immunity. It is not surprising that antimicrobial cellular immunity can be largely or completely divorced from delayed sensitivity, because this type of immunity depends on the direct effector activities of macrophages only, whereas delayed sensitivity and anti-tissue cellular immunity depend largely on the effector activities of lymphocytes.

A. Anti-tissue Cellular Immunity

Living cells and tissues which are recognized as foreign by host lymphoid elements stimulate an immune response. Although cells from a genetically dissimilar animal may persist and thrive in an immunologically deficient host, they are eliminated or rejected by a normal recipient. This emphasizes the well-established fact that rejection of foreign tissue is mediated by immunological mechanisms, rather than by the lack of a suitable environment for growth.

Tissues which behave as foreign are usually allogeneic or xenogeneic; they may even be "syngeneic" (male to female) or autologous. In the latter instance, they contain either occult antigens which accidentally reach immunologically competent cells, or autologous components with altered antigenicity. Autochthonous tumors arise from autologous tissues but contain new tumor-specific antigens which are foreign to the host.

The primary immunological response to cells or tissues recognized as foreign, which results in their rejection, depends largely on the specific activity of effector cells. Humoral antibodies alone are usually not sufficient to mediate rejection of primary allografts, even though they often figure prominently in rejection of xenografts and of second-set allografts. Although space does not permit a complete discussion of the mechanisms of graft rejection, excellent reviews are available (Billingham and Silvers, 1963; Russell and Monaco, 1964; Gowans and McGregor, 1965).

1. Allograft Immunity

The mouse skin allograft is a good model for studying cellular immunity to grafts. When a small skin graft is transplanted to an allogeneic recipient of a different H-2 genotype, it "heals in" during the first week in the same manner as an autograft. Grossly, the graft looks healthy for approximately 8 to 10 days before the first signs of rejection appear. These signs include ecchymoses, darkening, shrinking, loosening of the edges, and dryness. By about 10 to 15 days the graft resembles a scab and sloughs completely, leaving a denuded area which is soon covered by ingrowth of surrounding epithelium.

The events which lead to the rejection of an allograft have been studied extensively. Antigens from the graft reach the draining lymph nodes, chiefly via lymphatic vessels, and stimulate an immunological response. Macrophages evidently function in the afferent phase of the response by transporting or processing antigens, or both. This is indicated by the observations that either selective killing of macrophages with silica (Pearsall and Weiser, 1968a) or interference with their function (Brent and Medawar, 1961; Johnson, 1968) prior to grafting results in a modest but significant prolongation of allograft survival. Conversely, RES stimulation results in accelerated rejection of allografts (Halpern, Biozzi, and Stiffel, 1963; Wooles and DiLuzio, 1964). By 4 or 5 days after grafting some of the cells of the draining lymph nodes are immune, as evidenced by their ability to transfer specific immunity to a new host. The large pyroninophilic cells found in draining lymph nodes at this time represent a rapidly proliferating population of cells. They give rise to lymphocyte-like cells which leave the nodes in efferent lymph and reach the graft via the circulation. Circulating immune lymphocytes are largely responsible for graft rejection (Gowans and McGregor, 1965).

Mononuclear cells of varying sizes begin to infiltrate the graft site prior to any outward evidence of graft rejection; indeed, this infiltration is essential for graft rejection. However, the actual mechanism by which the immune cells cause destruction of the grafted cells remains a mystery. Electron microscopy has shown that the cell type which appears to function as the major effector of graft rejection is blast-like and has characteristics of both the lymphocyte and the macrophage (Wiener et al., 1964). It has been called by some an immature plasma cell (Kountz et al., 1963; Dempster, Harrison, and Shackman, 1964), and by others a macrophage (Binet and Mathé, 1962; Waksman, 1963). Large numbers of mature macrophages appear at the graft site as rejection proceeds. Although these macrophages are very much in evidence in the graft and graft bed, Dumonde (1967b) has proposed that they probably play no specific effector role in allograft rejection, but instead merely act as scavengers and possibly as processors of antigen. However, the evidence cited below indicates that macrophages may act as specific effector cells as well.

a. **Studies in Vivo.** Gorer (1958) noted that certain allografted tumors stimulate an abundant infiltration of macrophages into the tumor area, where they appear to contact and kill tumor cells following intimate asso-

ciation of the two types of cells. The tumor Sarcoma I (SaI) in the
C57BL/Ks (C57 black) mouse is one example. Others have been described, e.g. certain tumors of hamsters (Gershon, Carter, and Lane, 1967).
Weaver (1958) described the effector activities of macrophages in the
rejection of tumor allografts.

The SaI system has been a useful model for studying the mechanisms
of allograft rejection. This sarcoma originated as a chemically induced
tumor in an A-strain mouse. An appropriate intraperitoneal (i.p.) dose
of the tumor normally kills A/Jax mice within 10 days to 2 weeks; however, the same inoculum given to C57BL/Ks mice, either i.p. to cause
ascites tumor or subcutaneously (s.c.) to incite solid tumor growth, is
rejected as an allograft. These strains of mice differ at the strong H-2 locus.

Mitchison (1955) used the SaI system to demonstrate the passive transfer of allograft immunity with specifically sensitized lymph node cells.
Old *et al.* (1963) transferred immunity in the same system with peritoneal
exudate cells, rich in macrophages. Baker *et al.* (1962) made extensive
microcinematographic observations on peritoneal cells during the rejection
of ascites SaI tumor by C57 black mice. They noted that macrophages
made intimate contact with the allografted tumor cells; death of both cells
then occurred.

Subsequent studies showed that immune macrophages, collected from
C57 black mice at the peak of rejection of SaI tumor, were capable of
causing acute allogeneic disease (AAD) when transferred to the peritoneum of normal A/Jax recipients (Weiser *et al.*, 1965). Apparently the
immune macrophages reacted directly with target cells of the recipient
mice to cause extensive local injury and necrosis.

Later *in vivo* studies using the SaI system were reported by Tsoi and
Weiser (1967a, b), who confirmed the finding of Bennett (1965) that
allograft immunity to SaI can be passively transferred with purified
(>95%) preparations of immune peritoneal macrophages. Quantitative
protection tests in x-irradiated C57BL/Ks recipients showed that a ratio
of one macrophage to one tumor cell in the inoculum was sufficient to
inhibit tumor growth completely; indeed, a ratio of one macrophage to
as many as five tumor cells resulted in discernible inhibition of tumor
growth.

Other *in vivo* studies were conducted to determine whether immune
macrophages can function as effector cells in the rejection of normal skin
allografts (Pearsall and Weiser, 1968b). Earlier *in vitro* experiments,
some of which are discussed elsewhere in this chapter, had established that
C57BL/Ks macrophages, specifically immune to A/Jax antigens, can
destroy SaI tumor by a nonphagocytic contact mechanism independent of
C'. In order to determine whether this rejection mechanism might also
be effective against allografts of normal A/Jax skin placed on C57BL/Ks

mice, immune macrophages were transferred to both irradiated and non-irradiated recipients of skin grafts. Suspensions of purified well-washed SaI-immune peritoneal macrophages (95 to 98% macrophages) were placed directly on the graft bed immediately before transplanting the graft. Control animals given nonimmune macrophages, or immune macrophages trypsinized in a manner known to remove cytophilic antibodies from their surfaces, rejected their grafts normally. In contrast, untreated immune macrophages caused a highly significant acceleration of graft rejection. The possibility that the small numbers of lymphocytes contaminating the macrophage suspensions were the sole agents responsible for accelerated graft rejection was ruled out by control experiments using lymphocytes separated from the same peritoneal cell suspension.

In other experiments, attempts were made to alter graft rejection by using silica as a macrophage toxin to deplete the graft recipients of macrophages (Pearsall and Weiser, 1968a). The results indicated that macrophages can act as effector cells in rejection of allografts of normal tissue. When silica treatment was given at appropriate intervals prior to grafting, extensive macrophage destruction was observed and the survival of allografts of either SaI tumor or A/Jax skin was significantly prolonged. Silica treatment initiated as late as 6 days after grafting, when graft rejection was in progress, also resulted in a significant prolongation of graft survival. These results, in conjunction with the passive transfer studies discussed above (Pearsall and Weiser, 1968b), strongly suggest that the macrophage can contribute as a specific effector cell to the rejection of allografts of either normal tissue or tumor cells.

On the basis of these studies, Pearsall and Weiser (1968a, b) hypothesized (1) that macrophages contribute to the afferent phase of the allo-immune response, by transporting and processing antigens; (2) that later during the response macrophages adsorb and become "armed" with cytophilic antibodies produced by neighboring lymphoid cells; and (3) that such armed macrophages act as effector cells to aid in the destruction of grafted cells. It is evident that lymphocytes may perform several effector functions in graft rejection: one, the direct effector function of killing cells of the graft by contact mechanisms; another, the indirect function of producing cytophilic antibodies for arming macrophages; and in addition, they may produce other factors which contribute to the rejection process. It is probable that rejection of primary allografts results largely from the combined effector activities of immune lymphocytes and macrophages, the macrophages being specifically immune only by virtue of cytophilic antibodies synthesized by other cells.

b. Studies *in Vitro*. A number of *in vitro* models of alloimmune cell-target cell interactions have been described (see review by Turk, 1967). Although in many of these models the lymphocyte is used as the immune cell, in others the macrophage is employed. Granger and Weiser (1964, 1966) showed that mouse peritoneal macrophages collected during the peak of rejection of allografted SaI ascites tumor are capable of destroying target cells in culture. When immune macrophages are placed at loci on monolayers of specific target fibroblasts, they adhere to the target cells and mutual destruction of both types of cells occurs within 24 to 48 hours, resulting in the formation of plaques of clearing in the monolayers. The specificity of this reaction depends on cytophilic antibody on the macrophage surface. This antibody can be eluted by heating the macrophages at $56°$ C for 30 minutes. When the antibody is removed by trypsinization, the immune macrophages remain viable but are no longer effective as aggressor cells unless rearmed by exposure to heat-eluted cytophilic antibody.

The mechanisms of cell destruction in the immune macrophage-target cell interaction are not clear. Since there is no C' in the medium, C' lysis is improbable. It is known that some macrophages synthesize components of C'; thus it is possible that the immune macrophages synthesize or carry components of C' which contribute to cell destruction. Nevertheless, this is probably not the principal mechanism of destruction because the ultrastructural changes detected by EM are not characteristic of C' damage (Chambers and Weiser, 1969).

McIvor (1969) has discovered a specific macrophage cytotoxin (SMC) which is released from immune macrophages during the first 2 to 4 hours of contact with specific target cells. This agent, which is heat-labile ($56°$ C, 1 hour) and specifically cytotoxic for target cells, could account for target cell destruction accompanying the interaction of target cells with immune cells; however, this has not been established conclusively. Later in the interaction of immune macrophages and target cells a nonspecific cytotoxin is liberated which resembles the lymphocyte cytotoxin of Granger and Williams (1968). Electron microscope studies of immune macrophage-target cell interaction indicate that the macrophage may pinch off and engulf projecting portions of target cell membrane (Chambers and Weiser, 1969). This could also lead to target cell injury and death.

An additional mechanism which may be important in target cell killing is the change in membrane charge and permeability which often follows cellular interactions. Ambrose (1967) noted that addition of a positively charged polymer to an isolated membrane causes a reduction in the net charge, and subsequent contraction of the membrane. When there is a high net charge on the membrane the component charges repel each other resulting in membrane expansion. When the net charge is reduced, contraction of the membrane occurs. Changes in permeability caused by expansion or contraction of the membranes of cells in contact

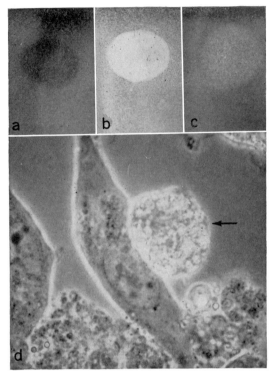

FIGURE 12-1. Adherence and destruction of specific target cells by alloimmune macrophages. The background areas (*a*) and (*b*) are stained monolayers of specific target fibroblasts which were overlaid at a central locus with alloimmune macrophages. The central dark spot in area (*a*) represents macrophages which have adhered specifically to target cells after five minutes. The clear plaque in area (*b*) is devoid of interacting cells which have undergone death and lysis (twenty-four hours). The background monolayer in area (*c*) was composed of a mixture of equal numbers of specific target cells and "nonspecific" cells. Hence, the central area of macrophage overlay is only partially cleared because only specific target cells have been killed. A high power field of early immune macrophage-target cell interaction (four hours) is shown in area (*d*). The arrow points to an immune macrophage filled with clear lipid droplets in contact with the dark target fibroblast. Note that the macrophage has compressed the cytoplasm of the target cell. (Mag. × 1250.) (Courtesy of K. L. McIvor.) (From Weiser, Myrvik, and Pearsall: "Fundamentals of Immunology." Lea & Febiger, Philadelphia, 1969.)

could be the basis of cell death resulting from immune cell-target cell interaction.

2. Immunity to Autochthonous Tumors

Although for many years immunity to autochthonous tumors was considered to be nonexistant, the work of Foley (1953), which was confirmed and extended by Prehn and Main (1957), established that a highly specific cellular immunity may be operative against such tumors. Much of the pertinent literature has been reviewed by Alexander and Fairley (1963), Smith (1968), and Hellström and Hellström (1969).

Tumor immunity is primarily a cellular immunity which operates in much the same manner as allograft immunity. Because tumors grow rapidly it has been proposed that they outgrow or overwhelm the immune forces of the host and consequently flourish even in the face of an active immune response.

It is probable that tumors oppose the immune forces of the host by the interaction of several mechanisms (see review of Hellström and Hellström, 1969). Among numerous possibilities are the following: (1) the tumor cell may produce a coating of sialomucin, or other substances, which protects against immune forces; (2) the massive amounts of antigen produced by the rapidly growing tumor may incite a state of immunological paralysis or tolerance; and (3) enhancing antibodies which interfere with cellular immunity may be synthesized by the host.

Lymphocytes play the major effector role in cellular immunity to autochthonous tumors, but it is possible that macrophages also perform effector functions. There is evidence suggesting that macrophages are important in the effector phase of immunity against certain chemically induced tumors; Old, Boyse, Bennett, and Lilly (1963) demonstrated that macrophage-rich preparations of peritoneal cells from animals immunized with a tumor could transfer specific immunity to syngeneic recipients. An

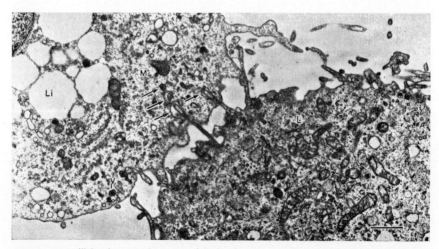

FIGURE 12-2. "Membrane phagocytosis" in immune macrophage-target cell interaction. Surface projections of an L cell (L) extend into invaginations of the lipid (Li)-containing macrophage (M) and appear to be undergoing phagocytosis (↗). A virus particle (V), from the L cell, has apparently been phagocytized. Magnification: 8,700. (From Chambers and Weiser: Cancer Res. 29:312, 1969.)

observation made many years ago by Murphy (1926), and subsequently verified by others (see review by Alexander and Fairley, 1963), was that nonspecific stimulation of macrophages by RES-stimulating agents frequently results in increased resistance to autochthonous and other types of tumors.

3. Autoimmune Diseases

As suggested earlier, a cellular immunological response against altered or occult antigens of self appears to be the chief basis of autoimmune diseases. MacKay and Burnet (1963), Turk (1967), and Miescher and Müller-Eberhard (1968) have discussed many aspects of autoimmune disease in detail.

Waksman (1960) showed that during the development of experimental autoimmune orchitis, lymphocytes and macrophages infiltrate seminiferous tubules and appear to destroy spermatocytes.

In 15 of several hundred patients with male infertility, large numbers of macrophages were demonstrated in the semen (Phadke and Phadke, 1961). The origin of these cells is uncertain; however, they were actively phagocytizing and disposing of spermatozoa. Autoantibodies were demonstrated in a few of these patients, but their role in the pathogenesis of the disease was not evident. Autoantibodies cytophilic for macrophages may have contributed to the process; however, this possibility was not investigated.

The histopathological picture in experimental allergic encephalomyelitis is similar to that in other autoimmune diseases, with lymphocytes and macrophages infiltrating the target area (Waksman, 1959; Patterson, 1968). The histopathology of these autoimmune diseases is similar to that described for skin allograft rejection (see review by Rose, 1965).

The initiation of autoimmunity appears to depend primarily on lymphocyte activities. Although macrophages are conspicuous in the lesions of many autoimmune diseases, their exact role in these circumstances is uncertain. They undoubtedly serve as scavenger cells, but, in addition, may function as immune effector cells.

4. Theoretical Aspects of Anti-tissue Cellular Immunity

It is reasonably certain that both immune lymphocytes and macrophages, carrying antibodies on their surfaces, can act as effector cells in anti-tissue cellular immunity. These surface antibodies, which cause specific adherence of immune cells to target cells, are synthesized by the lymphocytes which carry them but are adsorbed as cytophilic antibodies by macrophages.

The effector activities of immune cells may depend, not only on surface antibodies, but also on other properties of the cells. Immune macrophages adhere to target cells by virtue of a specific reaction between macrophage-cytophilic antibodies and target antigens; however, cell destruction results from other properties of the macrophage. This is clearly shown by experiments in which the specific effector activity of immune macrophages is lost when the cells are depleted of cytophilic antibody by trypsin treatment, and is restored by exposure to cytophilic antibody; in contrast, normal or nonspecifically immune macrophages do not gain effector activity simply by acquiring specific cytophilic antibodies (Weiser *et al.*, 1969).

The properties of immune macrophages which account for the actual destruction of target cells have not been defined. The killing of target cells may result from action of the heat-labile specific cytotoxin liberated by macrophages early in the interaction, or by other mechanisms, such as phagocytosis of bits of target cell membrane, or changes in electric charge on membranes.

The mechanisms of destruction of target cells by immune lymphocytes are also unknown. Cell destruction could result from the action of the nonspecific heat-stable cytotoxin which is liberated late in the cellular interaction. This lymphocyte cytotoxin may contribute to anti-tissue cellular immunity in ways other than by a direct cytotoxic action on target cells. It could induce normal lymphocytes to undergo blast transformation and to liberate more cytotoxin; in addition, it could attract, immobilize, and activate macrophages in the vicinity of the graft. Immune lymphocytes probably also contribute to anti-tissue cellular immunity by synthesizing antibodies cytophilic for macrophages.

Recent investigations into the nature of the cytotoxic factors formed by lymphocytes and macrophages during delayed sensitivity reactions and immune cell-target cell interactions may help to elucidate the relation between delayed sensitivity and anti-tissue cellular immunity.

B. Antimicrobial Cellular Immunity

Antimicrobial cellular immunity has been discussed extensively in a number of recent reviews (Mackaness and Blanden, 1967; Turk, 1967; Dannenberg, 1968); in this chapter attention will be centered on macrophage function in antimicrobial cellular immunity.

The role of macrophages in virus infections has been discussed by Mims (1964a), who reviewed the literature concerning clearance of virus particles from the circulation by cells of the RES, the influence of macrophage activity on host susceptibility to infection by viruses, and virus-macrophage interaction. Macrophages phagocytize virus particles and either support their growth, allow their survival until they are passed to other cells, or destroy them. In the last event, virus antigen may be conserved for stimulating the immune response, or the virus particle may be completely degraded; viruses coated with specific antibodies are especially prone to digestion by the macrophages that they normally infect. In the case of vaccinia virus, antibody interferes with the escape of the virus from the phagosome into the cytoplasm of the host cell, and thereby prevents viral replication.

Except for viruses and rickettsiae, most intracellular pathogens are limited to macrophages. This probably obtains for two principal reasons: first, because macrophages are phagocytic, and, second, because macrophages are cells which live long enough to allow ample time for intracellular parasites to multiply. In contrast, other phagocytes, such as PMNs, do not harbor intracellular parasites for extended periods because they are short-lived cells. The phagocytic activity of both PMNs and macrophages is required for total protection of the host, inasmuch as PMNs can engulf but do not destroy certain organisms, e.g. *M. tuberculosis,* which are effectively controlled only by macrophages, and, conversely, certain microbes are more effectively destroyed by PMNs than by macrophages. Apart from phagocytosis, PMNs may act in other ways to supplement the activity of macrophages. For instance, Rebuck, Whitehouse, and Noonan (1967) have described a process of glycogen transfer from PMNs to macrophages, which normally aids in macrophage metabolism. In addition, the homeostatic interactions between PMNs and macrophages, discussed in Chapter 5, could profoundly affect the macrophage response.

Although cellular immunity may be invoked by a wide variety of intracellular microorganisms, including viruses, mycological agents, and animal parasites, the response to bacteria has been the most studied.

In general, the effector mechanisms of cellular immunity are weaker and slower acting than are those of humoral immunity. This accounts in part for the chronicity of the diseases which are controlled by cellular immunity. These infections are caused by organisms which are not susceptible to acquired humoral factors or which are protected from humoral factors because their intracellular habitat affords them shelter. In order to multiply intracellularly, these organisms must be able to resist the antimicrobial forces within macrophages and to meet their growth needs within this microenvironment. Many microbes fail in these respects, and consequently are readily destroyed following phagocytosis by macrophages.

Macrophages can be activated, either specifically or nonspecifically, by many foreign materials, including bacterial products; following activation they demonstrate an increased capacity to inhibit or destroy a wide variety of intracellular organisms. Nonspecific activation of macrophages can be caused by nonantigenic microbial products, such as endotoxins and other lipids. Specific activation has been shown to follow the reaction of antibodies with antigens of the macrophage membrane, resulting in a greatly increased rate of pinocytosis and formation of enzymes by the macrophage (Cohn and Parks, 1967c). It is probable that antibodies cytophilic for macrophages can activate the macrophage in a similar manner, by reacting with foreign antigen reaching the cell surface.

The capacity of different macrophages to suppress ingested bacteria is determined, to some measure at least, by the degree of activation of the cell at the time of encounter with the microbe, i.e. the higher levels of enzymes in activated, as compared with nonactivated, macrophages (Heise, Myrvik, and Leake, 1965; Mizunoe and Dannenberg, 1965; Saito and Suter, 1965). For example, most normal alveolar macrophages are moderately activated and are more effective than immature blood monocytes in suppressing microbes. This does not imply that nonactivated macrophages are unable to cope with ingested microorganisms, for the ingested organisms themselves commonly stimulate rapid activation of the host cells.

In antimicrobial cellular immunity, macrophage activation and increased resistance appear to result from the stimuli provided by specific immunological events, in combination with nonspecific stimuli. This concept is supported by several observations: first, the time of appearance of immune macrophages following primary challenge with the organism is characteristic of an immunological response; second, an anamnestic accelerated response of activated macrophages follows a secondary challenge; and, finally, a number of conditions which depress immunological capability also depress the activated macrophage response of cellular immunity. It is also well established that activated macrophages persist only as long as the antigenic stimulus is present, suggesting that specific activation is maintained by frequent or continuous stimulation, demanding both cytophilic antibody and antigen.

The nature of the infecting organism is a crucial factor in determining the effectiveness of cellular immunity, both at the local site of infection and systemically. In mouse typhoid, in which the infection causes extensive necrosis, immunity may be less effective locally than systemically (Mackaness, Blanden, and Collins, 1966), presumably because necrosis leads to a *locus minoris resistentiae*. On the other hand, tuberculosis in rabbits can result in a cellular immunity which is more marked and persistent at the local site than systemically (Dannenberg *et al.,* 1968). Although macrophages in many areas may be activated as a result of the systemic dissemination of soluble antigens, a higher degree of activation occurs at the site of infection, not only because of exposure to high concentrations of antigens, but also because nonantigenic lipids, waxes, or other particulate and insoluble microbial products which stimulate nonspecifically tend to remain at infected foci.

Macrophages which have been highly active in phagocytizing and killing intracellular organisms frequently mature into epithelioid cells, and finally fuse to form giant cells within granulomas. The epithelioid cell probably represents the ultimate in antimicrobial resistance (Pernis *et al.,* 1966; Dannenberg, 1968). Phagocytized bacteria can be seen within activated macrophages, but are usually completely degraded by the time that the epithelioid cell stage of maturation is reached; microorganisms are seldom seen in epithelioid cells, even though many lysosomes are present. As a rule, giant cells contain neither engulfed material nor large numbers of lysosomes.

Intracellular inhibition or destruction of bacteria is influenced by a number of environmental factors. For example, virulent *Salmonella typhimurium* is destroyed to a greater extent by normal macrophages than by macrophages from vitamin-deficient rats (Furness and Axelrod, 1959). As another example, cigarette smoke has been shown to depress the intracellular killing of *Staphylococcus albus* by cultured rabbit alveolar macrophages (Green and Carolin, 1967). Obviously, factors in the microenvironment of the macrophage may alter this cell's capacity to develop and express cellular immunity.

The models that have been most used to study antibacterial cellular immunity are infections with mycobacteria, listeriae, salmonellae, and a number of other intracellular pathogens. Each of these model systems will be discussed below.

1. Mycobacterial Systems

a. Tuberculosis. A discussion of the early work on cellular immunity in tuberculosis has been presented by Lurie (1964). Lurie and Dannenberg (1965) reviewed studies on macrophage function in tuberculosis using strains of rabbits inbred for either resistance or susceptibility to the disease. They considered resistance to be primarily a function of host macrophages. A comparison of the macrophages of susceptible and resistant strains of rabbits indicated that resistance to primary infection with tubercle bacilli is influenced by two functions of host macrophages, namely phagocytosis and early intracellular inactivation of the organisms. The alveolar macrophages of resistant rabbits were much more efficient in phagocytizing and inactivating tubercle bacilli than were those of susceptible rabbits. The evidence reviewed clearly demonstrates that the capabilities of macrophages determine the progress of tuberculous infections. Even before infection, macrophages from resistant rabbits contain much higher levels of enzymes, e.g. dehydrogenases and acid phosphatase, than are found in macrophages from susceptible rabbits. Following infections in resistant strains of rabbits, the macrophages of these animals become able to inhibit markedly the multiplication of the bacilli. Macrophages of infected resistant rabbits mature more rapidly to epithelioid cells in the lesions than do macrophages from susceptible rabbits, and *in vitro* they are more resistant to the cytotoxic effects of tubercle bacilli than are macrophages of susceptible rabbits.

In addition, Lurie and Dannenberg (1965) reported that rabbits became highly susceptible to tubercle bacilli following thyroidectomy or treatment with antithyroid drugs or cortisone. The bacilli proliferated more readily in treated than in untreated animals, and maturation of macrophages to epithelioid cells was delayed in the treated animals. The reverse was true in rabbits made hyperthyroid; in these animals proliferation of the organisms was slowed and maturation of macrophages to epithelioid cells was speeded. Alteration of either adrenal or thyroid function altered the numbers of macrophages which could be obtained from the peritoneum and caused changes in enzyme levels of the macrophages, indicating that both the numbers available and the state of activation of macrophages are important in cellular immunity. Evidently the capacity of macrophages to engulf and destroy or suppress the growth of tubercle bacilli depends on the genetic potential of the host and on factors which influence gene expression, e.g. hormones.

Hsu and Kapral (1960) allowed immune peritoneal macrophages from guinea pigs to phagocytize tubercle bacilli *in vitro* and then cultured them for periods as long as 12 days. As compared to normal macrophages, multiplication of the organisms within the immune macrophages was greatly retarded.

In their studies on the interaction between tubercle bacilli, antibodies, and macrophages, Fong *et al.* (1956, 1957) used trypsinized macrophages from either nonimmune or immune animals, incubated with either nonimmune or immune serum. Immune serum protected both nonimmune and immune macrophages against the cytotoxicity of the organisms. The inhibition of multiplication of the bacilli within activated immune macrophages was largely nonspecific. Antibacterial activity was manifested to varying degrees against a variety of other intracellular bacteria. Elberg (1960) suggested that antibodies in immune serum contribute importantly to cellular immunity to tuberculosis by protecting immune macrophages from the toxic effects of tubercle bacilli.

Similarly, Hsu (1965) demonstrated that normal macrophages from susceptible rabbits are more vulnerable to the cytotoxic effects of virulent tubercle bacilli than are immune macrophages; immune macrophages can also restrict the intracellular growth of the organisms. Moreover, immune serum protected these normal macrophages against the cytotoxic effects of virulent organisms. It was postulated that resistance of immune cells to cytotoxic damage might result from the activity of cytophilic antibodies on immune macrophages.

Youmans and Youmans (1969) have reviewed their extensive investigations, and the work of others, on the nature of acquired immunity to tuberculosis. By the use of living cells of a strain of *M. tuberculosis* that did not multiply in the mice being studied, they established that live organisms are hundreds of times more effective for producing immunity than are heat-killed organisms. They also demonstrated that tubercle bacilli contain two immunogens. One immunogen is a heat-stable component of the cell wall, possibly a lipopolysaccharide, that immunizes equally well against *M. tuberculosis* and nonrelated organisms such as *L. monocytogenes*. The other immunogen is a labile ribosomal component which, when incorporated in Freund's incomplete adjuvant, immunizes specifically against *M. tuberculosis*. The mycobacterial ribosomes contain protein and RNA. Their immunogenicity is inactivated by treatment with RNAase but not with trypsin. Since digestion with pronase was not tried, the possibility that the immunogen is a complex containing a protein, or protein fragment and RNA, was not ruled out. The ribosomal immunogen did not incite delayed sensitivity to ribosomal protein or to tuberculin. Youmans and Youmans pointed out that the immunogen may be RNA complexed to some low molecular weight component which could act as a super-antigen in the manner of a macrophage-processed antigen; it could induce immunity by inciting an antibody to RNA (which could inhibit intracellular multiplication of tubercle bacilli) or alternatively by inciting macrophages to produce a growth-inhibiting substance, such as an adaptive enzyme.

The granulomatous response, characteristic of tuberculosis and many other chronic infectious diseases, can be induced specifically by antigens and nonspecifically by such agents as silica and the nonantigenic cord factor of *M. tuberculosis*. Kawata, Myrvik, and Leake (1964) showed that a specifically induced accelerated response can be elicited by administering tubercle bacilli i.v. to a BCG-vaccinated rabbit. This accelerated granulomatous response is independent of tuberculin sensitivity. It may possibly be caused by antigen-stimulated proliferation of macrophages bearing cytophilic antibodies.

Since the macrophage is the principal agent of resistance to tuberculosis, it is reasonable to expect that the activated macrophages of granulomas should afford more immunity against intracellular parasites than nonactivated macrophages can provide, regardless of the stimulus responsible for the granuloma. The work of Youmans and Youmans (1969) strongly supports this concept. These investigators showed that resistance of vaccinated mice to early specific challenge with virulent *M. tuberculosis* is directly correlated with the extent of the granulomatous response induced by the vaccine. Protection was most pronounced when the challenge inoculum was given by a route which permitted the organisms to reach the granulomatous tissue induced by the vaccine. The design of the experiment was such that the resistance measured was probably independent of the antibody response and rested principally with macrophages which were exercising immunity gained through nonspecific activation by bacterial components.

In order to study the specificity of acquired cellular immunity, Coppel and Youmans (1969) vaccinated mice with *L. monocytogenes* or with viable attenuated *M. tuberculosis.* Weeks afterwards, groups of animals were given booster doses of the respective vaccines. Twenty-four hours later the following groups of mice were challenged with a virulent strain of *L. monocytogenes:* those vaccinated only, those vaccinated and boosted, those not vaccinated, and those given a "booster" dose only. At daily intervals ranging from 3 to 7 days, spleens were removed and the numbers of viable organisms were estimated by plate counts. With respect to anti-listeria immunity, the results indicated that (1) immunity induced with both vaccines waned to essentially zero at the time of challenge but could be reestablished anamnestically with specific vaccine, (2) both vaccines induced low but significant early immunity in some nonspecific manner, and (3) a specific anamnestic response to the challenge organism became clearly evident on the third day following challenge.

b. **Leprosy.** Leprosy is an unusual disease with respect to the different courses it takes and the wide variety of lesions it presents. Indeed, leprosy could prove to be the most complete model of the granulomatous diseases. Its study promises to contribute greatly to an understanding of the mechanisms of cellular immunity.

Although the causative agent of leprosy, *Mycobacterium leprae,* was discovered almost a century ago, the organism has not been cultivated in non-living media and is extremely difficult to propagate in normal experimental animals. It is an intracellular parasite, and could be either facultative or obligatory since it is uncertain whether it can grow extracellularly. Shepard (1960) succeeded in producing mild self-limiting infections in the mouse footpad, and Rees and co-workers (1967) have obtained extensive infections in mice crippled immunologically by a combination of thymectomy and x-irradiation.

Little is known about the factors which determine variation in the immunity of different animal species to a given microbe. In leprosy, it would seem reasonable that the unique susceptibility of the human species might lie in certain intrinsic properties of the human macrophage, which simultaneously enable it to support the nutritional needs of *M. leprae* but prohibit it from acquiring the capacity to inhibit or destroy the organism. Since the ability of an animal to respond to a given antigenic determinant may be genetically determined, the defect responsible for susceptibility to leprosy could be a genetic incapacity to respond to important antigens of the organism. This would not be unexpected, because genetic defects in PMN capabilities have been shown to result in a chronic granulomatous disease (Holmes, Page, and Good, 1967), and it is reasonable to assume that comparable genetic defects occur in macrophages.

The extent of immunity to leprosy in man is probably determined not only by inherent properties of the macrophage, but also by other immune forces, perhaps contributed by lymphocytes, which act together with the macrophages. The finding that immunologically crippled mice with extensive and progressing leprosy rapidly regain effective immunity following receipt of syngeneic immunocompetent lymphoid cells by passive transfer (Rees, 1968) emphasizes the fact that in this disease the immunological activities of lymphocytes must contribute significantly to the antibacterial cellular immunity expressed by effector macrophages.

The high susceptibility of the lepromatous patient to leprosy may be considered to rest in part on a species defect and in part on an individual defect. However, no clues are presently available to indicate whether the defect(s) is in the macrophage and/or the antibody-producing cells, or elsewhere.

Leprosy is a chronic disease which resembles tuberculosis in many ways. The organisms in local lesions gain entrance into the blood with relative ease and are transported to sites of elective localization in low-temperature areas of the body. *Mycobacterium leprae* probably has an optimum growth temperature below 37° C, since it multiplies preferentially in low-temperature areas. The organism has a predilection for nerves, especially those exposed to trauma. The bacilli in lesions are virtually all confined within macrophages and Schwann cells. The observation of Rees and associates (1967) that *M. leprae* grows abundantly in striated muscle cells of immunologically depressed mice indicates that macrophages and Schwann cells are not the only cells capable of satisfying the growth requirements of *M. leprae* and emphasizes the question of why the organisms do not grow readily in cultured cells.

The two polar forms of the disease are lepromatous leprosy, in which granulomas fail to develop and extensive multiplication of organisms occurs, and tuberculoid leprosy, in which typical granulomas develop and multiplication of organisms is limited. Intermediate forms of the disease occur and may ultimately convert to either of the two polar forms.

Skin tests are of value for determining the form of leprosy, because tuberculoid and lepromatous patients exhibit different responses to antigens of *M. leprae*. The test most often used employs killed *M. leprae* (lepromin) obtained from human lesions. These whole, killed bacilli may elicit an early delayed sensitivity type of response to bacillary proteins (the Fernandez reaction) or may engender a granulomatous response which becomes apparent weeks later (the Mitsuda reaction). Less frequently, an extract of bacillary proteins is used to test for delayed sensitivity only.

Tuberculoid leprosy is characterized by a marked resistance to the bacilli. Few bacilli are found in the granulomatous lesions, which are rich in epithelioid cells and are encompassed by a dense zone of lymphocyte infiltration (Ridley and Jopling, 1966). Patients with tuberculoid leprosy react to the lepromin test with both the early Fernandez and the late

Mitsuda reactions, and also give a positive delayed sensitivity reaction to bacillary proteins alone.

By contrast, lepromatous leprosy is characterized by a lack of immunity to the organisms. The lepromatous lesions are composed of macrophages containing enormous numbers of bacilli. The granulomatous response is conspicuously absent; epithelioid cells and lymphocytes are lacking in the lesions. Antibodies to bacillary carbohydrates are abundant in the serum, but both cellular immunity and delayed sensitivity to *M. leprae* are depressed. The delayed sensitivity reaction to soluble bacillary proteins is usually negative. These patients also have little or no capacity to respond to the lepromin test with either the early Fernandez or the late Mitsuda reaction.

The bases of the reactions to antigens of *M. leprae,* in normal or infected individuals, are not fully apparent or clearly understood. Whereas early reactions to soluble protein antigens reflect an existing state of delayed sensitivity to these antigens, late reactions to lepromin are more complex and reflect a capacity to react to whole organisms with granulomatous response. This granulomatous response could include two components: one, an allergic response to antigens of the organisms, and the other, a nonallergic response to nonantigenic bacillary constituents.

The significance of the lepromin reaction in man has been discussed by Rees (1964). If it is assumed that the primary granulomatous response to lepromin reflects the capacity to respond, rather than a preexisting state of sensitivity, most normal individuals would be expected to give positive Mitsuda lepromin reactions. Reactions to lepromin in normal individuals vary from near zero in infants to 90% in adults. This finding suggests that the capacity to respond to lepromin is acquired with age, but whether this has an element of acquired sensitivity or is solely a physiological change with age is not evident. It has been suggested that the capacity to respond to lepromin is a reflection of the ability of the macrophages to digest the bacilli (Beiguelman and Barbieri, 1965); it was observed that the macrophages of lepromin-positive, but not lepromin-negative, patients were able to digest the bacilli. This observation has been extended to include lepromin-positive and lepromin-negative normal individuals of different ages (Barbieri and Correa, 1967).

Beiguelman and Qualgliato (1965) presented evidence to support the concept that the marked capacity of macrophages to lyse *M. leprae* and to mount the lepromin reaction is hereditary. There may be an analogy between this situation in man and the behavior of either live or killed *M. leprae* in the macrophages of guinea pigs and rats, as observed by Hadler and associates (see literature citation by Hadler, Ferreira and Ziti, 1965). These investigators have reported that, whereas guinea pig macrophages are able to lyse *M. leprae* and transform into epithelioid cells to form typical granulomas, rat macrophages do not lyse the injected organisms, but, instead, store the organisms and fail to transform to epithelioid cells.

The concept proposed is that lysis of *M. leprae* provides granulomagenic materials, both antigenic and nonantigenic, which incite the lepromin reaction; because the macrophages of lepromin-negative individuals lack the capacity to lyse the bacilli, the granulomatous response is not stimulated. This important concept demands additional investigation to determine its validity.

There is other evidence which indicates that the capacity to mount a granulomatous response to lepromin predetermines the ability to resist *M. leprae*. In a study by Dharmendra and Chatterjee (1955), reviewed by Rees (1964), lepromin tests were performed on 680 healthy individuals in a rural area where leprosy was endemic. It was found that 524 were lepromin-positive and 156 were lepromin-negative; 16 remained negative despite repeated lepromin tests. Reexamination 15 to 20 years later revealed that 17 of the 524 who were initially lepromin-positive had acquired leprosy, but all 17 had developed the tuberculoid form of the disease. On the other hand, 15 of the 156 lepromin-negative persons had acquired leprosy, and over half of these had the lepromatous type of the disease. Moreover, 10 of the 16 who initially remained negative to repeated lepromin tests acquired leprosy, and all 10 developed the lepromatous form of the disease. These data provide a strong indication that, even in healthy subjects, the capacity to respond to lepromin is a measure of resistance to leprosy and that failure to respond, especially to repeated lepromin tests, predicts an increased chance of acquiring leprosy and of developing the lepromatous form of the disease.

The lack of an existing state of delayed sensitivity to extracts of *M. leprae* in lepromatous leprosy may be due in some measure to generally depressed capacity either to develop this type of sensitivity or to mount a delayed reaction; nonetheless, the reason for failure of the lepromatous patient to develop delayed sensitivity to lepromin is chiefly specific. Recently it has been shown that a limited degree of delayed sensitivity to lepromin, as measured by the Fernandez reaction at 48 hours, can be transferred to lepromatous patients with buffy coat cells from tuberculin sensitive normal subjects (Paradisi, de Bonaparte, and Morgenfeld, 1969).

A moderately lowered capacity to develop allergic responses of the delayed type is often noted in lepromatous leprosy. Waldorf *et al.* (1966) and Bullock (1968) have demonstrated that lepromatous patients have a defect in the ability to develop delayed sensitivity to contact allergens. Dierks and Shepard (1968) also noted that the capacity of lymphocytes from untreated patients with lepromatous leprosy to undergo blast transformation on exposure to either PHA or antigens of *M. leprae* or *M. tuber-*

culosis is depressed. In contrast, the depression was considerably less in drug-treated lepromatous patients and those with tuberculoid leprosy. Bullock (1968) reported that the lymphocytes from lepromatous patients have a lowered capacity to respond to either PHA or specific antigen with blast transformation and DNA synthesis. The work of Paradisi, de Bonaparte, and Morgenfeld (1968) has provided confirmatory evidence that the PHA response is depressed in patients with lepromatous leprosy. Sheagren *et al.* (1969) observed that in lepromatous patients, IgA and IgG serum levels are high, the RES is hyperactive, and lymphocyte blast transformation in response to streptolysin O is depressed.

It has also been reported that a nonspecific humoral factor which inhibits lymphocyte blast transformation by PHA is present in the serum of some lepromatous patients (Bullock, 1968). Such an agent could account for the failure of these patients to mount delayed sensitivity reactions, which appear to depend on lymphocyte blast transformation. Other evidence of a defective immune response in lepromatous leprosy is provided by the observation of Han and Weiser (unpublished results) that lepromatous patients have a lessened capacity to reject skin allografts; this capacity is almost normal in tuberculoid patients. It appears that the abilities of lepromatous patients to respond specifically to *M. leprae* with delayed sensitivity, granuloma formation, and cellular immunity are completely suppressed; however, there is usually only a partial suppression of these patients' capacity to respond to other bacteria, to reject skin allografts, to exhibit lymphocyte blast transformation, to express delayed sensitivity to tuberculin, and to develop delayed sensitivity to contact allergens. The observation that some of these immunological defects ameliorate as the disease improves with treatment strongly supports the concept that such nonspecific defects are primarily the result of the disease, rather than a cause. The fact that they occur to a lesser degree in tuberculoid patients than in lepromatous patients is consistent with this view.

The strong correlation between depression of specific delayed sensitivity and the lack of effective cellular immunity in lepromatous leprosy, and the presence of specific delayed sensitivity and effective cellular immunity in tuberculoid leprosy, suggests that the two phenomena are interrelated. However, direct evidence to support this concept is lacking. In lepromatous leprosy, specific depression of delayed sensitivity and cellular immunity to *M. leprae* could result from immunological tolerance, immunological enhancement, or immune deviation; whereas nonspecific suppression of these phenomena could result from competition of antigens, cytotoxic effects of the organisms, or other causes.

The phenomenon of immunological enhancement, described in tumor and transplantation systems (see reviews by Kaliss, 1958, 1965, 1966; Hellström and Möller, 1965), deserves to be investigated in relation to antimicrobial cellular immunity. Immunological enhancement is defined as enhanced survival of incompatible tissue grafts caused by specific humoral antibodies. A similar interference with cellular immunity against microorganisms might occur, and contribute significantly to the development of the lepromatous state in leprosy and comparable states in other diseases.

The range of immunopathology between the tuberculoid and lepromatous forms of the disease is most marked in leprosy; however, a similar range has been observed in a number of other diseases that are controlled by cellular immunity. Examples are coccidioidomycosis, histoplasmosis, and leishmaniasis, in which the disease may be restricted by the granulomatous reaction, as in tuberculoid leprosy, or may be characterized by disseminated, progressive disease, high titers of serum antibodies, and lack of delayed sensitivity and true granuloma formation, as in lepromatous leprosy. Thus, the studies on mechanisms of infection and host response, so clearly demonstrated in leprosy infections, are applicable to a large group of diseases.

2. The Listeria System

Listeria monocytogenes is a motile gram-positive rod, which usually exists within macrophages; therefore the host depends on cellular immune mechanisms to control the infection. An outstanding characteristic of this organism is the marked monocytosis which it engenders. A lipid component of the organism, termed "monocytosis-producing agent" (MPA), can be extracted and can also incite the monocytogenic response (Stanley, 1949, 1950; Holder and Sword, 1969).

Cellular immunity to listeriosis in mice was discussed in a review by Mackaness (1968). It has been reported that, within 4 days after infection, *L. monocytogenes* can incite an immunity capable of protecting mice against 10^4 lethal doses of virulent listeria (Mackaness, 1962). This immunity can be passively transferred with cells but not with serum (Miki and Mackaness, 1964), and is accompanied by a state of delayed sensitivity to the organisms (Mackaness, 1962).

The effectiveness of passive transfer of cellular immunity to listeria with macrophages may depend on the availability of transferred macrophages to the challenge dose of bacteria. In passive transfer experiments, macrophages from mice convalescing from *L. monocytogenes* infections are highly effective in suppressing a challenge dose of the organisms, provided both macrophages and bacilli are administered intraperitoneally.

The observation that specific immunity can be transferred with purified preparations of immune lymphocytes given intravenously (Mackaness, 1968) clearly indicates that lymphocytes contribute in some way to cellular immunity, and ultimately to destruction of organisms by macrophages.

The lymphocyte contribution could be an antibody, probably one which serves as a macrophage-cytophilic antibody. Such antibody might activate the macrophage upon contact with antigen; alternatively, it could protect the macrophage against toxic effects of the organisms or aid in their intracellular destruction. Although lymphocytes participate in the central immune response, it should be reemphasized that macrophages are the only cells which can act directly as the effector in antimicrobial cellular immunity because they are the cells which must contact, phagocytize, inhibit, and destroy the microbes.

3. The Salmonella System

Conflicting evidence has been obtained concerning the importance of humoral antibodies in immunity against salmonella infections. Rowley, Turner, and Jenkin (1964) have maintained that cytophilic antibody contributes to immunity to salmonella infections; others have expressed the view that cellular immunity is largely independent of humoral influences. Mackaness and co-workers (1966) found that transfusion of immune serum did not affect the course of salmonella infection in mice. They also showed (Blanden et al., 1966) that washed macrophages from salmonella-infected mice or listeria-infected mice display notably enhanced microbicidal properties, as compared with macrophages from noninfected mice. Moreover, these macrophages killed either salmonellae or listeriae, even though no cross-reacting humoral antibodies could be demonstrated, suggesting that serum antibodies are not essential for effective cellular immunity.

Jenkin and Rowley (1963) reviewed some of the literature on immunity to typhoid in mice. They concluded that cytophilic antibodies on the surfaces of macrophages are responsible for the macrophages' ability to recognize particles as foreign and to express bactericidal activity.

Turner, Jenkin, and Rowley (1964) studied the molecular characteristics of the antibodies formed by mice infected with *S. typhimurium*. The peak titers of 19S antibody in serum occurred 14 days after a single dose of viable attenuated *S. typhimurium,* and decreased steadily thereafter; while the 7S antibody titer increased from day 14 to day 42. Rowley, Turner and Jenkin (1964) demonstrated that the capacity of immune peritoneal macrophages to transfer immunity to *S. typhimurium* in mice is due to the presence of 19S cytophilic antibody which can be eluted from the cells. At a time when 19S antibody levels decrease, the immune capacities of peritoneal macrophages also decline. Trypsinization of the macrophages to remove or destroy cytophilic antibodies partially abrogates their capacity to transfer immunity. Moreover, normal macrophages acquire a degree of immunity when they are trypsinized and then exposed to serum containing specific cytophilic antibodies. Rowley and co-workers also passively transferred immunity to *S. typhimurium* in mice with large amounts of 14-day immune serum (presumably rich in 19S antibodies) given over a 3-day period prior to challenge with opsonized virulent organisms (Jenkin, Rowley, and Auzins, 1964). Thus, in this system, cytophilic 19S antibodies appear to play a major role in cellular immunity.

There are other reports that, in mice, immunity to salmonella infections can be passively transferred with macrophages (Saito *et al.*, 1962).

4. Other Antimicrobial Systems

Other antimicrobial systems in which cellular immunity seems to be of primary importance include infections with *Pasteurella sp., Brucella sp.,* certain viruses, animal parasites, and mycological agents (see reviews by Elberg, 1960; Suter and Ramseier, 1964; Mackaness and Blanden, 1967).

It was clearly shown by Pomales-Lebron and Stinebring (1957) that *Br. abortus* can multiply within normal guinea pig macrophages *in vitro.* However, cultured immune peritoneal macrophages were able to destroy the organisms or suppress their growth.

These findings were confirmed and extended by Holland and Pickett (1958) who showed that, whereas *Br. abortus, Br. suis,* and *Br. melitensis* can multiply extensively within cultured macrophages of the normal mouse, rat, or guinea pig, restricted growth of the organisms occurred within macrophages from animals previously infected with the particular species of brucella. The addition of specific antiserum to the culture medium had no effect on intracellular growth of the bacteria in this system.

Holland and Pickett (1958) also showed that guinea pigs infected with living, smooth *Br. suis* give positive delayed skin reactions to brucellergen, while guinea pigs vaccinated with heat-killed, smooth *Br. suis* develop high titers of agglutinating antibodies, but do not develop demonstrable delayed sensitivity to brucellergen. Although vaccination with living, rough *Br. suis* also induced a state of delayed sensitivity to smooth brucella antigen, the monocytes from these guinea pigs were not capable of inhibiting intracellular growth of the bacteria. Thus, in these experiments, cellular immunity could be induced only with living, smooth brucellae but was effective against both smooth and rough variants. The results suggested that, in brucella infections, delayed sensitivity is not directly related to cellular immunity.

In a different system using *Br. melitensis* and cultured rabbit macrophages, Ralston and Elberg (1969) demonstrated that immune serum confers upon both immune and normal macrophages an increased capacity to adhere to, phagocytize, inhibit, and kill the organisms. They showed that immune macrophages can resist the necrotizing effects of virulent organisms and can accomplish some initial killing and restriction of bacterial growth, but that these antimicrobial effects continue only in the presence of immune serum. They stressed the possibility that an interaction between macrophages and immune serum may be necessary in order for macrophages to express their full immunological potential. Cytophilic antibodies, by reacting with antigen of the infecting organisms, may provide a metabolic stimulus to macrophages, resulting in an increased capacity to ingest, kill, or restrict intracellular growth of the organisms.

The influence of immune serum on the intracellular fate of brucellae appears to vary with the experimental system used. Fitzgeorge, Solotorovsky, and Smith (1967) reported that, in a bovine system, *Br. abortus* multiplies more slowly in immune macrophages than in nonimmune macrophages, but immune serum has no effect on intracellular multiplication of the bacteria in either case. They also noted that the PMNs of normal cattle are more destructive for *Br. abortus* than are the macrophages.

The participation of macrophages and other cell types in immunity to infections with animal parasites was discussed in a review by Soulsby (1967). Although humoral antibodies against animal parasites may often be demonstrated (Smithers, 1967), many of these parasites, e.g. *Leishmania sp.,* commonly live within macrophages where they are protected from humoral influences. Following infection with *Leishmania tropica,* macrophages proliferate locally and afford a site for intracellular multiplication of the parasite. Over a period of several months, lymphocytes and plasma cells infiltrate the area; macrophages simultaneously cease proliferating and decrease in numbers; the number of parasites also decreases and the lesion disappears (Adler, 1963). The resulting immunity, established only after the cellular events described have occurred, may last for as long as two decades. Interruption of the cellular events by excision of cutaneous lesions abrogates immunity and leaves the host susceptible to reinfection (Adler, 1963).

Infections with animal parasites may occur in some individuals without inciting a lymphoid cell response or a delayed skin reaction to antigens of the parasite. For instance, *Leishmania tegumentaria diffusa* occasionally grows freely within macrophages of the host, apparently unopposed. It has not been determined whether this condition is due to the genetic constitution of the host or to some property of the parasite, or both (Adler, 1963). Animals such as gerbils, which are reservoirs for the parasites, also exhibit extensive macrophage proliferation and intracellular growth of the organism with relatively slight lymphoid cell infiltration into infected areas.

Phagocytosis by macrophages plays a major role in the pathogenesis and in the course of some infections due to animal parasites. For example, in malaria there is a marked erythrophagocytosis, not only of infected red cells but also of uninfected cells (Cox, Schroeder, and Ristic, 1965). Malarial parasites within macrophages may be eliminated from the blood stream via the bronchial tree (Bilbey, Cox, and Nicol, 1963). Various explanations have been offered for the increased phagocytic activities of the RES during parasitic infections, as reviewed by Soulsby (1967); however, the mechanisms involved are not clearly defined. It is conceivable that lipids of the parasites act to stimulate phagocytosis, or that cytophilic antibodies or antigen-antibody complexes may be involved. As yet, macrophage-cytophilic antibodies directed against antigens of animal parasites have not been demonstrated, but it is reasonable to suppose that they occur.

Immunity to animal parasites can be transferred with cells (Dineen and Wagland, 1966; Larsh, 1967; Dineen, Wagland, and Ronai, 1968). In view of the variety of animal parasites and the complexity of their life cycles, it is to be expected that they would incite a great diversity of immune responses, both cellular and humoral. Nevertheless, the many animal parasites which live within mammalian macrophages are controlled largely by cellular immune mechanisms.

5. Ultrastructural Responses of Macrophages to Intracellular Microbes

Electron microscopy has revealed several patterns of intracellular response of macrophages to various microbes. These responses depend on the virulence of the organisms and on the degree of resistance of the host macrophages.

A frequent response to the ingestion of bacteria within phagosomes is the usual formation of phagolysosomes, with the subsequent digestion of the organisms. This pattern has been observed in mouse peritoneal macrophages within an hour after the ingestion of *L. monocytogenes* (North and Mackaness, 1963a), in human macrophages from patients with tuberculoid leprosy (Imaeda, 1965), and in many other infections.

Less frequently, virulent organisms produce toxic substances which may affect the integrity of phagosomal membranes. Armstrong and Sword (1966) found that some macrophages from mice infected with *L. monocytogenes* contained bacilli in contact with the cytoplasm. It was suggested that virulent listeria may release a lysin with lecithinase or phospholipase activity, resulting in lysis of areas of host cell membrane. A similar observation was made by Njoki-Obi and Osebold (1962), who noted the lysis of peritoneal exudate cells of sheep infected with *L. monocytogenes*. It has been proposed that cytophilic antibodies coating macrophage surfaces can remain attached during phagocytosis and consequently line the phagosomal membrane; in this position they may oppose the destructive effects of bacterial toxins on the phagosomal membrane or other structures. Such a mechanism could allow the survival of activated macrophages over periods of time sufficient for them to destroy phagocytized microorganisms.

Other patterns of macrophage response to ingested bacteria are observed, often following the disruption of phagosomal membranes. Mycobacteria engulfed by macrophages may become enclosed within laminated structures formed by deposition of new membrane. Leake and Myrvik (1966) described the appearance of phagocytized *M. smegmatis* tightly encased in multilaminated structures which appear to be phagosomes enclosed within membranes that have been laid down in a sequential manner. Another response is the fusion of the membranes of several lysosomes to form "giant lysosomes" which engulf whole phagosomes containing tubercle bacilli (Dumont and Sheldon, 1965). In still other instances, lysosomes adhere to phagosomes but fail to fuse and discharge their contents in the normal manner. Instead, lysosomal materials, apparently of low solubility, remain adherent to the bacilli at the point of contact between lysosomes and the phagosome, without demonstrable intervening membranes (Myrvik, personal communication). It has been postulated that certain mycobacteria which are not killed or inhibited within phagolysosomes may actually utilize lysosomal products as nutrients (Brown, Draper, and Hart, 1969). In this situation, rather than harm phagocytized bacilli, lysosomal enzymes may provide an additional source of substances essential for bacillary growth.

Enormous numbers of *M. leprae* are found in the macrophages of patients with lepromatous leprosy (Imaeda, 1965). These microorganisms may grow within phagosomes until the membranes are ruptured by physical stress or toxic effects. Often they lie free in the cytoplasm, where they grow and form large aggregates. At this time, an almost electron-transparent substance lacking acid phosphatase activity begins to accumulate around the bacilli and appears to fuse with the cytoplasm of the macrophage. It was postulated that it represents an accumulation of bacterial metabolites. Gradually a membrane is formed around the bacillary clump

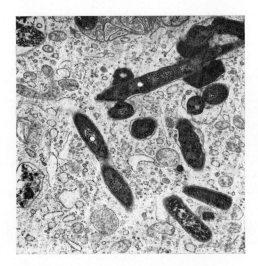

FIGURE 12-3. Alveolar macrophage from a nonimmunized rabbit injected intratracheally with living *Mycobacterium smegmatis* 24 hours before the micrograph was taken. The intracellular organisms show little change in morphology. The peribacillary space in the phagosome is minimal or absent. Magnification: 11,000. (Courtesy of E. S. Leake and Q. N. Myrvik.)

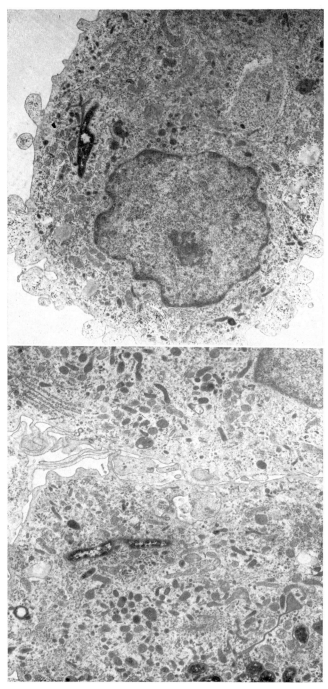

FIGURE 12-4. Alveolar macrophages from rabbits injected intratracheally with living *M. smegmatis* 5 days before the micrographs were taken. At this time the mycobacteria show some cytoplasmic degeneration. A peribacillary space is lacking. Magnification: 9,300. (Courtesy of E. S. Leake and Q. N. Myrvik.)

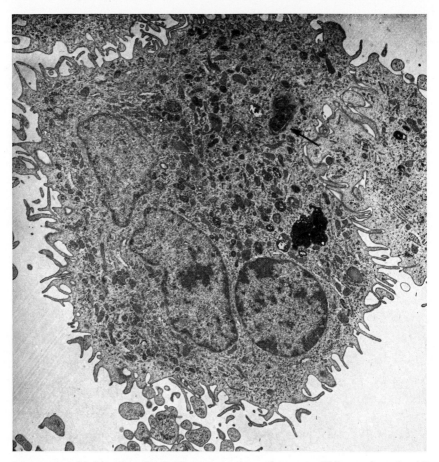

FIGURE 12-5. Multinucleated alveolar macrophage from a rabbit vaccinated with killed BCG 3 weeks before the micrograph was taken, and given an intratracheal injection of living *M. smegmatis* 3 hours before the cells were collected. Within the huge, highly activated cell, mycobacteria can be seen in vacuoles. Activated cells commonly show a deposit of electron-dense material surrounding the phagosome (arrow). Magnification: 6,200. (Courtesy of E. S. Leake and Q. N. Myrvik.)

and associated substance. In the macrophages of lepromatous lesions there are other membrane-bound structures typical of phagolysosomes, containing bacilli and acid-phosphatase-positive, dense, granular substance. These structures occur more often in drug-treated than in untreated lepromatous patients. With time, phagolysosomes may become filled with degenerating bacilli and are then highly vesiculated.

Even in the lesions of lepromatous leprosy, many bacilli are dead and resemble empty shells devoid of cytoplasm. In acid-fast preparations they show irregular staining, as contrasted to live cells which are solid-stained rods. Obviously, even within the macrophages of lepromatous lesions, growth of the organism is not totally unrestrained. Whether limitation of growth is due to acquired resistance on the part of the macrophage, to exhaustion of nutrients, or to some other cause is not known.

6. The Relation of Delayed Sensitivity to Antimicrobial Cellular Immunity

The possible relation of delayed sensitivity to cellular immunity has long been a controversial subject. Because cellular immunity and delayed sensitivity are frequently associated, a causal relationship has been postulated (Mackaness and Blanden, 1967). Turk (1967), who has reviewed much of the evidence on this subject, concluded that the changes in macrophages which occur at the time when delayed sensitivity develops are chiefly responsible for cellular immunity, and that cellular immunity is unrelated to the inflammatory component of delayed sensitivity reactions. Rich (1951b) was one of the principal proponents of the concept that delayed sensitivity is basically harmful in tuberculosis. Others have taken the view that it is beneficial, at least under some circumstances. There is ample evidence that strong immunity to tuberculosis can exist without delayed sensitivity to tuberculin, and vice versa. Convincing proof of this is provided by the work of a number of investigators, e.g. Youmans and Youmans (1969), who produced strong immunity to tuberculosis with a ribosomal vaccine which does not induce delayed sensitivity, and Raffel (1961), who demonstrated that tuberculin hypersensitivity can exist in the absence of effective immunity to tuberculosis.

Thus, delayed sensitivity may not be essential for cellular immunity; however, it seems likely that it could contribute significantly to such immunity in some circumstances.

7. Theoretical Aspects of Antimicrobial Cellular Immunity

The mechanisms which account for the specificity of cellular immunity are the subject of much controversy. Theoretically, there are two components of the specificity of acquired cellular immunity: this immunity is specifically induced, and it can exhibit some specificity in its operation, i.e. in the effector activity of macrophages. The specificity of cellular immunity indicates that antibodies must participate at some point in the response. Jenkin and Rowley (1963) reviewed the role of antibodies in cellular immunity. They suggested that the activity of cell-bound or cytophilic antibodies may be of primary importance in this type of immunity. In addition to their classical role of promoting phagocytosis, antibodies have been implicated in the intracellular killing of certain bacteria by macrophages. The mechanisms involved are not known (Jenkin, 1963).

The specificity of the effector activities of macrophages, as observed by Coppel and Youmans (1969), could result from increased metabolic activity of the specifically activated cells. Alternatively it could result from the activity of cell-associated antibodies; such antibodies could lead to proliferation of antigen-stimulated macrophages, or could protect phagosomal membranes from the cytotoxic action of microorganisms, as discussed previously. In addition, the specificity of macrophage activity in cellular immunity may rest, in part, on the control of enzyme production by the available substrate. For example, the high lipid content of mycobacteria suggests that high concentrations of certain lipases may be effective in combating intracellular bacilli. Cells containing high concentrations of such enzymes produced in response to mycobacterial infection might well be more effective against mycobacteria than against brucellae or other bacteria containing various other substrates. This difference in enzyme levels within immune macrophages could confer a specificity to intracellular disposition of organisms, totally independent of antibody activity.

Mackaness and Blanden (1967) reviewed evidence which supports the concept that IgM cytophilic antibodies act as mediators of both anti-tissue and antimicrobial cellular immunity, and probably of delayed sensitivity as well. The possible role of cytophilic antibodies in antimicrobial cellular immunity has also been discussed by Weiser, Myrvik, and Pearsall (1969).

Since passive transfer of cellular immunity with serum has been reported only rarely, strongly cytophilic antibodies must usually be lacking from the serum but present on cell surfaces. Instead it is possible that antibodies with the strongest cytophilic properties are acquired by macrophages through direct contact with the lymphocytes that produce them. Even if macrophage-cytophilic antibodies are present in transferred serum, two characteristics of their activity may preclude their effectiveness in normal recipients. First, cytophilic antibodies exist in equilibrium between the cell-bound and free state and compete for cytophilic sites on macrophages. These sites on recipient macrophages may be saturated with cytophilic antibodies of other specificities, so that effective quantities of passively transferred antibodies cannot be adsorbed. Second, and perhaps more important, is the time required for macrophage activation following any stimulus, including a reaction between cytophilic antibodies and antigen at the cell surface. The macrophages of the recipient may not be sufficiently activated at the time of transfer to withstand the challenge, even if aided by cytophilic antibodies. It is possible that the occasional report of success in passively transferring cellular immunity with serum rests on fulfilling the following conditions: (1) high concentrations of strongly cytophilic antibodies were transferred; and (2) activated macrophages were abundant in the host and available to the transferred cytophilic antibodies.

The observation that lymphocytes, as well as macrophages, can transfer cellular immunity, is not inconsistent with the concept that macrophage-cytophilic antibodies mediate cellular immunity. Since lymphocytes probably form cytophilic antibodies, transferred lymphocytes could provide a source of continuing cytophilic antibody production.

Another finding which supports the probability that cytophilic antibodies are important in cellular immunity is that the extent of macrophage activation depends on the amount of antigenic stimulation. With large doses of infecting organisms, macrophages throughout the body may become activated, whereas with lower infecting doses the immunity tends to be localized at the focus of infection. If lymphocytes in close association with high concentrations of antigen in infected foci are the most active in producing cytophilic antibodies, macrophages in that area should become preferentially coated with such antibodies, and subsequently activated by reaction with antigens at the site. However, when antigen is abundant and escapes from the local area, macrophages throughout the body could become supplied with cytophilic antibodies produced elsewhere.

Additional pertinent observations are that macrophage activation persists only so long as the antigenic stimulus is present and that, after infection has terminated, cellular immunity wanes rapidly but can be quickly recalled on secondary challenge. If the reaction of antigen with cytophilic antibodies on macrophages provides an important stimulus for macrophage activation, it affords an explanation for these findings.

The evidence cited indicates that antibodies cytophilic for macrophages contribute significantly to cellular immunity. On the other hand, it is possible that their role is minor and that other mechanisms account for the observations discussed above. For instance, the accelerated specific anamnestic response could be associated with a delayed sensitivity reaction, i.e. sensitized lymphocytes could react specifically with antigen and release nonspecific factors responsible for the accumulation and activation of macrophages. Both alternatives are logical enough to support the working hypothesis that cytophilic antibodies and lymphocyte factors contribute to cellular immunity by complementing each other. More evidence is required to support or deny this hypothesis conclusively.

SUMMARY: The term "acquired cellular immunity" is used to define that immunity which results from the effector activities of cells and which can be transferred with cells but not with serum. Both anti-tissue and anti-microbial cellular immunity share certain general characteristics, and differ in some respects.

In most types of acquired cellular immunity, macrophages function in the transporting and processing of foreign antigens during the afferent phase of the immunological response. Macrophages also fulfill their scavenger functions in the various kinds of cellular immune responses. In addition, an effector function has been ascribed to immune macrophages during the rejection of allografts and probably during the response to autochthonous tumors.

Activated macrophages are essential for the expression of antimicrobial cellular immunity because the parasites are destroyed or inhibited within these cells. Macrophages may be activated by both specific and non-specific mechanisms. The role of cytophilic antibodies in cellular immunity and the possible relation of delayed sensitivity to cellular immunity are considered. Although delayed sensitivity is not essential for cellular immunity, it could contribute; it is postulated that lymphocytes may act as effector cells or may synthesize antibodies that are cytophilic for macrophages, and in both ways may contribute to cellular immunity. In addition, during delayed sensitivity reactions, lymphocytes synthesize and release substances which may cause the chemotaxis of macrophages, their immobilization at the site of antigen, and perhaps their activation. Overall, lymphocytes and macrophages cooperate in an effective cellular immune response.

Chapter 13
Macrophages in Disease

THE PARTICIPATION of macrophages in cellular immunity against a number of chronic infectious diseases has been discussed in Chapter 12. Macrophages also play a prominent role in the pathogenesis and course of other diseases.

Perhaps the most readily recognized abnormality involving macrophages is monocytosis, i.e. an increase in the proportion, or occasionally in the absolute number, of monocytes in the blood. Normally, monocytes constitute 3 to 8% of the leukocytes of peripheral blood, but the percentage of monocytes may be as high as 90% during certain infections and neoplastic states. Bacterial infections which commonly result in monocytosis include tuberculosis, brucellosis, typhoid fever, and subacute bacterial endocarditis (SBE). Infections with certain protozoa and rickettsiae also lead to monocytosis.

A. Infectious Diseases

In addition to their essential role in the pathogenesis of granulomatous diseases, macrophages can play a prominent role in other infectious diseases. For example, substantial numbers of mature macrophages are sometimes observed in the peripheral blood of patients with SBE. Daland *et al.* (1956) reviewed this subject and reported a number of cases. Macrophages are more easily demonstrable in ear lobe blood, because the ear lobe is a dependent low-temperature area where circulating cells tend to accumulate. More than 10% of the leukocytes in the first drop of blood from an ear lobe puncture of patients with SBE may be macrophages. Greenberg (1964) reported a patient in whom mature macrophages constituted 32% of the leukocytes in the first drop of ear blood collected after puncture; ear lobe blood of this patient contained 8 to 40 times as many macrophages as venous blood. There was a good correlation between the response of the patient to antibiotic therapy and decreasing macrophage counts.

The tendency for circulating macrophages to accumulate in the ear lobe may also account for the reported success in demonstrating acid-fast bacilli (presumably *M. leprae*) in ear lobe blood (S. H. Han, personal communication) of patients with lepromatous leprosy.

The increased susceptibility of diabetic patients to infection may be related to a failure of the usual mechanism for transfer of glycogen from PMNs to macrophages (Rebuck, Whitehouse, and Noonan, 1967). Normally, glycogen is transferred from neutrophils to macrophages and apparently is utilized as an energy source for macrophage activities. Although the transfer of glycogen to macrophages was substantial in inflammatory foci of normal subjects, it was greatly suppressed in patients with severe diabetes, particularly during post-acidotic periods.

B. *Metabolic Diseases*

The role of macrophages in the pathogenesis of atherosclerosis has been reviewed by Day (1967). The deposits of lipid found in the intima of atherosclerotic arteries result, at least in part, from macrophage activity. The composition of these lipids indicates that they are not simply deposited by filtration, but instead are metabolic products, probably derived from macrophages in the arterial wall. Fat-laden macrophages (foam cells) are abundant in early atherosclerotic lesions, and play an active role in the metabolism of lipids in the lesions.

Other abnormalities of lipid metabolism are also associated with unusual changes in macrophages. Histiocytosis X is a generic term used to designate a group of diseases of unknown etiology in which xanthomatous granulomas are the distinguishing characteristic. Eosinophilic granuloma, Letterer-Siwe disease, and Schüller-Christian disease are included in the general category of Histiocytosis X (Avioli, Lasersohn, and Lopresti, 1963). These diseases progress through four stages: (1) a phase of macrophage proliferation and accumulation of eosinophils, (2) a vascular-granulomatous phase, during which macrophages and eosinophils persist and small collections of lipid-laden macrophages form, (3) a diffuse xanthomatous phase, during which many foam cells accumulate, and (4) in chronic cases, a final phase of healing and fibrosis.

An unusual rodlike tubular body has been found in macrophages of patients with Histiocytosis X (deMan, 1968). Although these bodies are probably related to the disease process, their origin and nature are unknown. It is postulated that they may represent either nonspecific cytoplasmic products which react in some way during the disease, storage of some organic products such as lipids, or some infective agent such as a virus.

Gaucher's disease is characterized by lipid accumulations within greatly enlarged macrophages; however, the glycolipids found in these (Gaucher) cells are glucocerebrosides containing equimolar amounts of sphingosine, fatty acid, and glucose (Moore, 1967). The disease is a rare familial autosomal recessive disorder, apparently caused by deficiency of an enzyme necessary for the degradation of certain glycolipids.

Another example of a hereditary lipidosis is the hypercholesterolemia that is transmitted as an autosomal dominant trait. In this disease, nodular masses of macrophages containing lipids, called xanthomas, are found in the skin and tendons (Walter and Israel, 1963).

C. Intercellular Imbalances

Pulmonary diseases characterized by unusual macrophage activity are numerous, and usually involve an imbalance in the normal interrelationship of cells in the lung. They include diffuse interstitial pulmonary fibrosis (Ebert, 1967), endogenous lipoid pneumonia (Maier, 1967), idiopathic pulmonary hemosiderosis (Christie, 1967a), and the pneumoconioses (Christie, 1967b). Fibrosing alveolitis, which precedes pulmonary fibrosis, is commonly associated with hyperfunction of macrophages. The relation between macrophages and fibroblasts has been discussed in Chapter 5. It is clear that destruction of mature macrophages is associated with fibrosis.

A desquamative interstitial pneumonia has been described; in this disease masses of large PAS-positive cells accumulate in the alveolar spaces, accompanied by an infiltration of lymphocytes and plasma cells (Liebow, Steer, and Billingsley, 1965). A model closely approximating this disease has been produced in rabbits by i.v. injection of Freund's complete adjuvant (Deodhar and Bhagwat, 1967). It was proposed that both the human disease and the animal model represent a hypersensitivity reaction in the lungs. Both respond well to treatment with steroid hormones.

A rapidly fatal form of silicosis has been described by Buechner and Ansari (1969), who reported four cases of acute silico-proteinosis in sandblasters. In each case, the patient had been exposed to large quantities of extremely small particles of silica over the relatively short period of 3 to 6 years. After onset of symptoms the average survival was only 7.5 months before the patients died with an acute alveolar proteinosis. It is possible that this form of acute silicosis results from a prolonged massive destruction of alveolar macrophages by large quantities of inhaled minute particles of silica; that this involves a compensatory proliferation with huge numbers of alveolar macrophage being continuously formed and rapidly destroyed; and that the destroyed macrophages release the proteinaceous material which fills the alveoli. It is probable that the lack of granulomatous foci typical of chronic silicosis can be attributed to the continuous and rapid proliferation of immature macrophages which are overwhelmed by the large quantity of silica and destroyed before granuloma formation can take place.

Abnormal activities of macrophages and certain macrophage-like cells occur in rheumatic diseases. The lining cells of synovial membranes are classified as Type A, macrophage-like phagocytic cells, and Type B, fibroblast-like cells with a rich endoplasmic reticulum. Electron microscopy of synovia from patients with rheumatoid arthritis reveals proliferation of Type A cells and the presence of many inclusions, containing a variety of ingested materials, within Type A cells (Norton and Ziff, 1966; Wyllie, Haust, and More, 1966). Lysosomal enzymes derived from PMNs, synovial lining cells, macrophages, and perhaps other types of cells are substantially increased above normal levels in rheumatoid synovial fluid (Weissman, 1966).

Certain anti-inflammatory agents, useful in the treatment of rheumatoid arthritis and other rheumatic diseases, are known to affect lysosomal stability and activity. Fedorko, Hirsch, and Cohn (1968) reported that colloidal gold is a membrane stabilizer. Persellin and Ziff (1966) demonstrated that gold salts, which are often used in treatment of rheumatic diseases, become concentrated in the lysosomes of guinea pig macrophages. It was further shown that gold salts inhibited the activities of lysosomal enzymes within these cells.

These and similar observations suggest that lysosomal enzymes of PMNs and macrophages participate in the pathogenesis of rheumatoid arthritis, gout, and pseudogout. The relative roles of various cell types in the pathogenesis of these diseases deserve intensive study.

D. Macrophages and Neoplasms

The literature on histiocytic neoplasms was reviewed by Braunsteiner and Gall (1962), who described the characteristics of various human neoplasms of reticuloendothelial tissue, and determined the enzyme content of both normal and neoplastic monocytes.

Neoplasms which cause monocytosis include monocytic leukemia, Hodgkin's disease, and the reticuloendothelioses (Leavell and Thorup, 1960). Dargeon (1966) made a clinical survey of the reticuloendothelioses of childhood.

Salm (1962) has proposed that the presence of collections of lipid-containing macrophages in endometrial lesions is strongly indicative that the lesions are malignant. Such macrophage collections were found in 10.8% (14 of 129) of patients having endometrial polyps, and in 7.5% (8 of 107) of patients with endometrial adenocarcinoma. Other investigators have also found collections of macrophages in association with adenocarcinoma of the uterus in approximately 10% of the patients reported (Harris, 1958; Krone and Littig, 1959; Scully and Richardson, 1961).

E. Possible Contributions of Macrophages to the Pathogenesis of Disease States

Salky, Mills, and DiLuzio (1965) measured the clearance of a test lipid from the blood stream of patients with various diseases characterized by immunological abnormalities. Enhanced RES activity was demonstrated in patients with either rheumatoid arthritis, rheumatic fever, or certain other diseases. The intravascular half-times of injected particulates were on the order of 4.0 minutes as compared with normal values of about 7.5 minutes. Because macrophages can contribute to antibody production by virtue of their phagocytic and digestive activities (see Chapter 9), it was proposed that the enhanced RES activity observed in the above-named diseases contributes to the pathogenesis of these diseases.

Böhme (1965) observed an increase in phagocytosis by the RES following the introduction of antigen into experimental animals. He suggested that the RES functions in the development of certain experimental autoimmune diseases by removing and modifying the antigens.

Macrophages produce an endogenous pyrogen which may be responsible for fever in diseases in which they are prominent in the lesions (Hahn et al., 1967). It was shown that peritoneal macrophages can produce a pyrogen with characteristics similar to those of the pyrogen produced by PMNs.

SUMMARY: Increased numbers of circulating immature macrophages are found during the course of a number of infectious diseases and neoplasms. This monocytosis probably represents a migration of newly formed macrophages to areas of inflammation. Mature macrophages are sometimes present in the peripheral blood of patients with subacute bacterial endocarditis, especially in the blood from the ear lobe.

Macrophage activity is important in atherosclerosis and other abnormalities of lipid metabolism. Granulomatous and fibrotic diseases of the lung also entail a high degree of macrophage activity. Rheumatic diseases are characterized by increased release of lysosomal enzymes from macrophages and other cells in the joints; lysosomal stabilizers are useful in therapy.

Macrophages may function in the pathogenesis of certain diseases. They may modify antigens in autoimmune states, and they can produce endogenous pyrogen which may contribute to the pathogenesis of many diseases.

Bibliography

1. Abramoff, P. and Brien, N. B. 1968. Studies of the chicken immune response. II. Biologic activity of spleen "immunogenic RNA." J. Immunol. *100*:1210-1214.

2. Acton, J. D. and Myrvik, Q. N. 1966. Production of interferon by alveolar macrophages. J. Bact. *91*:2300-2304.

3. Ada, G. L., Parish, C. R., Nossal, G. J. V. and Abbot, A. 1967. The tissue localization, immunogenic, and tolerance-inducing properties of antigens and antigen-fragments. Cold Spring Harbor Symp. Quant. Biol. *32*: 381-393.

4. Adinolfi, M., Gardner, B. and Wood, C. B. S. 1968. Ontogenesis of two components of human complement: β_{1E} and β_{1C-1A} globulins. Nature *219*:189-191.

5. Adler, F. L. Fishman, M. and Dray, S. 1966. Antibody formation initiated *in vitro*. III. Antibody formation and allotypic specificity directed by ribonucleic acid from peritoneal exudate cells. J. Immunol. *97*:554-558.

6. Adler, S. 1963. Immune phenomena in leishmaniasis. *In* "Immunity to Protozoa." (Eds. Garnham, P. C. C., Pierce, A. E., and Roitt, I.) Blackwell, Oxford. pp. 235-245.

7. Agricola, G. 1556. *De re Metallica*, transl. by Hoover, H. C. and Hoover, L. H., 1912. The Mining Magazine. Salisbury House, London.

8. Alexander, P. and Fairley, G. H. 1963. Cellular resistance to tumours. Brit. Med. Bull. *23*:86-92.

9. Allison, A. C., Harington, J. S. and Birbeck, M. 1966. An examination of the cytotoxic effects of silica on macrophages. J. Exp. Med. *124*:141-154.

10. Ambrose, E. J. 1967. Possible mechanisms of the transfer of information between small groups of cells. *In* "Cell Differentiation." (Eds. De Reuck, A. V. S. and Knight, J.) Ciba Fndn. Symposium. Little, Brown & Co., Boston. pp. 101-110.

11. Amos, H. E., Gurner, B. W., Olds, R. J. and Coombs, R. R. A. 1967. Passive sensitization of tissue cells. II. Ability of cytophilic anti-

body to render the migration of guinea pig peritoneal exudate cells inhibitable by antigen. Intern. Arch. Allergy *32*:496-505.

12. Andersen, H. and Matthiessen, M. E. 1966. The histiocyte in human foetal tissues. Its morphology, cytochemistry, origin, function and fate. Zeit. f. Zellforsch. *72*:193-211.

13. Antonini, F. M. 1967. Importance of aging in the relationships between the reticuloendothelial system and cholesterol transport. Adv. Exp. Med. Biol. *1*:404-412.

14. Antweiler, H. 1959. Verstärkte Antikörperreaktion durch vorausgehende Adsorption des injizierten Antigens an Quarz. Naturwissenchaften *46*:360.

15. Arakawa, T. and Spaet, T. H. 1963. *In vitro* inactivation of rabbit blood thromboplastin by macrophages. Proc. Soc. Exp. Biol. Med. *113*:71-73.

16. Argyris, B. F. 1968. Role of macrophages in immunological maturation. J. Exp. Med. *128*:459-467.

17. Armstrong, B. A. and Sword, C. P. 1966. Electron microscopy of *Listeria monocytogenes*-infected mouse spleen. J. Bact. *91*:1346-1355.

18. Aronson, M. 1963. Bridge formation and cytoplasmic flow between phagocytic cells. J. Exp. Med. *118*:1083-1088.

19. Aronson, M. and Elberg, S. S. 1962. Proliferation of rabbit peritoneal histiocytes as revealed by autoradiography with tritiated thymidine. Proc. Nat. Acad. Sci. *48*:208-214.

20. Asherson, G. L. 1967. Antigen-mediated depression of delayed hypersensitivity. Brit. Med. Bull. *23*:24-29.

21. Askonas, B. A. and Rhodes, J. M. 1965. Immunogenicity of antigen-containing ribonucleic acid preparations from macrophages. Nature *205*:470-474.

22. de Asúa Jiménez, F. 1927. Die Mikroglia (Hortegasche Zellen) und das retikulo-endotheliale System. Zeit. f. ges. Neurol. u. Psych. *109*:354-379.

23. Austen, K. F. and Cohn, Z. A. 1963. Contribution of serum and cellular factors in host defense reactions. I. Serum factors in host resistance. New Eng. J. Med. *268*:933-938; 994-1000.

24. Avioli, L. V., Lasersohn, J. T. and Lopresti, J. M. 1963. Histiocytosis X (Schüller-Christian disease): A clinicopathological survey, review of ten patients and the results of prednisone therapy. Medicine *42*:119-147.

25. Ayoub, E. M. and McCarty, M. 1968. Intraphagocytic β-N-acetylglucosaminidase. J. Exp. Med. *127*:833-851.

26. Baillif, R. N. 1960. Reaction patterns of the reticuloendothelial system under stimulation. Ann. N. Y. Acad. Sci. *88*:3-13.

27. Baker, P., Weiser, R. S., Jutila, J., Evans, C. E. and Blandau, R. J. 1962. Mechanisms of tumor homograft rejection; the behavior of Sarcoma I ascites tumor in the A/Jax and the C57B1/6K mouse. Ann. N. Y. Acad. Sci. *101*:46-62.

28. Ballantyne, B. 1967. Esterase histochemistry of reticuloendothelial cells. Adv. Exp. Med. Biol. *1*:121-132.
29. Balner, H. 1963. Identification of peritoneal macrophages in mouse radiation chimeras. Transplantation *1*:217-223.
30. Barbieri, T. A. and Correa, W. M. 1967. Human macrophage culture. The leprosy prognostic test (LPT). Intern. J. Leprosy *35*:377-381.
31. Barker, C. F. and Billingham, R. E. 1968. The role of afferent lymphatics in the rejection of skin homografts. J. Exp. Med. *128*:197-221.
32. Barnes, D. W. and Wooles, W. R. 1968. The effect of reticuloendo- thelial stimulation on pentobarbital metabolism. (Abstr.) J. Retic- uloendothel. Soc. *5*:22-23.
33. Barrow, J., Tullis, J. L. and Chambers, F. W., Jr. 1951. Effect of x- irradiation and antihistamine drugs on the reticulo-endothelial sys- tem measured with colloidal radiogold. Amer. J. Physiol. *164*: 822-831.
34. Bauer, H. 1968. Cellular defense mechanisms. *In* "The Germ-Free Animal in Research." (Ed. Coates, M. E., Assoc. Eds. Gordon, H. A. and Wostmann, B. S.) Academic Press, New York. pp. 210-226.
35. Beard, J. W. and Rous, P. 1934. The characters of Kupffer cells living *in vitro*. J. Exp. Med. *59*:593-607.
36. Beiguelman, B. and Barbieri, T. A. 1965. Compartamento dos macró- fagos nas formas polares da lepra. Ciência e Cultura *17*:304-305.
37. Beiguelman, B. and Quagliato, R. 1965. Nature and familial character of the lepromin reactions. Intern. J. Leprosy *33*:800-807.
38. Benacerraf, B. 1965. Delayed hypersensitivity. *In* "The Inflammatory Process." (Eds. Zweifach, B. W., Grant, L. and McCluskey, R. T.) Academic Press, New York. pp. 577-586.
39. Benacerraf, B. 1968. Cytophilic immunoglobulins and delayed hyper- sensitivity. Fed. Proc. *27*:46-48.
40. Benacerraf, B., Kivy-Rosenberg, E., Sebestyen, M. M. and Zweifach, B. W. 1959. The effect of high doses of x-irradiation on the phago- cytic, proliferative and metabolic properties of the reticulo-endo- thelial system. J. Exp. Med. *110*:49-64.
41. Bennett, B. 1965. Specific suppression of tumor growth by isolated peritoneal macrophages from immunized mice. J. Immunol. *95*: 656-664.
42. Bennett, B. 1966. Isolation and cultivation *in vitro* of macrophages from various sources in the mouse. Amer. J. Path. *48*:165-181.
43. Bennett, B. 1967. Comparative morphology of macrophages in tissue culture. Adv. Exp. Med. Biol. *1*:74-84.
44. Bennett, I. L., Jr. and Cluff, L. E. 1957. Bacterial pyrogens. Pharm. Rev. *9*:427-475.
45. Bennett, W. E. and Cohn, Z. A. 1966. The isolation and selected prop- erties of blood monocytes. J. Exp. Med. *123*:145-159.
46. Berken, A. and Benacerraf, B. 1966. Properties of antibodies cyto- philic for macrophages. J. Exp. Med. *123*:119-144.

47. Berken, A. and Benacerraf, B. 1968. Sedimentation properties of anti-body cytophilic for macrophages. J. Immunol. *100*:1219-1222.
48. Berman, I. 1967. The ultrastructure of erythroblastic islands and reticular cells in mouse bone marrow. J. Ultrastruct. Res. *17*:291-313.
49. Berman, L. 1966. Lymphocytes and macrophages *in vitro*. Their activities in relation to functions of small lymphocytes. Lab. Invest. *15*:1084-1099.
50. Berman, L. and Stulberg, C. S. 1962. Primary cultures of macrophages from normal human peripheral blood. Lab. Invest. *11*:1322-1331.
51. Berry, L. J. and Spies, T. D. 1949. Phagocytosis. Medicine *28*:239-300.
52. Bertalanffy, F. D. 1964. Respiratory tissue: Structure, histophysiology, cytodynamics. Part II. New approaches and interpretations. Int. Rev. Cytol. *17*:213-297.
53. Bessis, M. 1956. "Cytology of the Blood and Blood-forming Organs." Grune & Stratton, New York. 629 pp.
54. Bessis, M. 1963. Quelques données cytologiques sur le rôle du système réticulo-endothélial dans l'erythropoïese et l'erythroclasie. Colloques internationaux du C.N.R.S. *115*:447-457.
55. Bilbey, D. L. J., Cox, F. E. and Nicol, T. 1963. Elimination of *Plasmodium berghei* by way of the respiratory tract in mice. Trans. Roy. Soc. Trop. Med. Hyg. *57*:271-273.
56. Bilbey, D. L. J. and Nicol, T. 1963. The molecular basis of drug effect on R.E.S. activity. Colloques internationaux du C.N.R.S. *115*:109-121.
57. Billingham, R. E. and Silvers, W. K. 1963. Sensitivity to homografts of normal tissues and cells. Ann. Rev. Microbiol. *17*:531-564.
58. Binet, J. L. and Mathé, G. 1962. Optical and electron microscope studies of the immunologically competent cells during the reaction of graft against the host. Ann. N. Y. Acad. Sci. *99*:426-431.
59. Biozzi, G., Halpern, B. N., Benacerraf, B. and Stiffel, C. 1956. Phagocytic activity of the reticuloendothelial system in experimental infections. *In* "Physiopathology of the Reticuloendothelial System." (Eds. Halpern, B. N., Benacerraf, B. and Delafresnaye, J. F.) Charles C Thomas, Springfield, Ill. pp. 204-225.
60. Bisset, K. A. 1946. The effect of temperature on non-specific infections of fish. J. Path. Bact. *58*:251-258.
61. Bisset, K. A. 1947. Bacterial infection and immunity in lower vertebrates and invertebrates. J. Hyg. *45*:128-135.
62. Blanden, R. V. 1968. Modification of macrophage function. J. Reticuloendothel. Soc. *5*:179-202.
63. Blanden, R. V., Mackaness, G. B. and Collins, F. M. 1966. Mechanisms of acquired resistance in mouse typhoid. J. Exp. Med. *124*:585-600.
64. Blickens, D. A. and DiLuzio, N. R. 1965. Metabolism of methyl palmitate, a phagocytic and immunologic depressant, and its influence on tissue lipids. J. Reticuloendothel. Soc. *2*:60-74.
65. Bloom, B. R. and Bennett, B. 1966. Mechanism of a reaction *in vitro* associated with delayed-type hypersensitivity. Science *153*:80-82.

66. Bloom, B. R. and Bennett, B. 1968. Migration inhibitory factor associated with delayed-type hypersensitivity. Fed. Proc. 27:13-15.

67. Bloom, W. 1928. Mammalian lymph in tissue culture. From lymphocyte to fibroblast. Arch. Exptl. Zellforsch. Gewebezücht 5:269-307.

68. Bloom, W. 1938a. Lymphocytes and monocytes: Theories of hematopoiesis. In "Handbook of Hematology," v. I. (Ed. Downey, H.) Paul B. Hoeber, Inc., New York. pp. 374-435.

69. Bloom, W. 1938b. Fibroblasts and macrophages (histiocytes). In "Handbook of Hematology," v. II. (Ed. Downey, H.) Paul B. Hoeber, Inc., New York. pp. 1335-1374.

70. Bloom, W. 1948. "Histopathology of Irradiation from External and Internal Sources." McGraw-Hill, New York. p. 752.

71. Bloom, W. and Fawcett, D. W. 1962. "A Textbook of Histology," 8th edition. W. B. Saunders Co., Philadelphia. p. 102.

72. Boak, J. L., Christie, G. H., Ford, W. L. and Howard, J. G. 1968. Pathways in the development of liver macrophages: Alternative precursors contained in populations of lymphocytes and bone-marrow cells. Proc. Roy. Soc., Ser. B. 169:307-327.

73. Boggs, D. R. 1966. Homeostatic regulatory mechanisms of hematopoiesis. Ann. Rev. Physiol. 28:39-56.

74. Böhme, D. 1965. The influence of experimental allergic muscular dystrophy on the reticuloendothelial system. J. Reticuloendothel. Soc. 2:47-59.

75. Borel, Y., Fauconnet, M. and Miescher, P. 1967. Dissociation of immune responses by the induction of partial unresponsiveness. Relationship of PCA and complement-fixing antibody formation to the suppression of delayed hypersensitivity. J. Immunol. 98:881-887.

76. Bosworth, N. and Archer, G. T. 1962. A phagocytosis-promoting substance present in eosinophils. Aust. J. Exp. Biol. Med. Sci. 40:277-281.

77. Bowden, D. H., Davies, E. and Wyatt, J. P. 1968. Cytodynamics of pulmonary alveolar cells in the mouse. Arch. Path. 86:667-670.

78. Boyden, S. V. 1960. Antibody production. Nature 185:724-727.

79. Boyden, S. V. 1962. Cellular discrimination between indigenous and foreign matter. J. Theor. Biol. 3:123-131.

80. Boyden, S. V. 1963. Cytophilic antibody. In "Cell-bound Antibodies." Wistar Inst. Press, Philadelphia, pp. 7-14.

81. Boyden, S. V. 1964. Cytophilic antibody in guinea pigs with delayed type hypersensitivity. Immunology 7:474-483.

82. Boyden, S. V. and Sorkin, E. 1960. The adsorption of antigen by spleen cells previously treated with antiserum in vitro. Immunology 3:272-283.

83. Boyden, S. V. and Sorkin, E. 1961. The adsorption of antibody and antigen by spleen cells in vitro. Some further experiments. Immunology 4:244-252.

84. Bradley, T. R. and Metcalf, D. 1966. The growth of mouse bone marrow cells in vitro. Aust. J. Exp. Biol. Med. 44:287-300.

85. Braun, W. and Lasky, L. J. 1967. Antibody formation in newborn mice initiated through adult macrophages. Fed. Proc. *26*:642.

86. Braunstein, H., Freiman, D. G. and Gall, E. A. 1958. Histochemical study of enzyme activities of lymph nodes. I. The normal and hyperplastic lymph node. Cancer *11*:829-837.

87. Braunstein, H. and Gall, E. A. 1962. The cytologic and histochemical features of malignant lymphoma. Progr. Hemat. *3*:136-154.

88. Braunsteiner, H., Dienstl, F., Sailer, S. and Sandhofer, F. 1964. Lipase activity in leukocytes and macrophages. Blood *24*:607-615.

89. Braunsteiner, H. and Schmalzl, F. 1968. Etude cytochimique des monocytes. Mise en évidence d'une estérase caractéristique. Nouv. Rev. Fr. d'Hémat. *8*:289-292.

90. Brecher, G., Endicott, K. M., Gump, H. and Brawner, H. P. 1948. Effects of X-ray on lymphoid and hemopoietic tissues of albino mice. Blood *3*:1259-1274.

91. Brent, L. 1958. Tissue transplantation immunity. Progr. Allergy *5*:271-348.

92. Brent, L. and Medawar, P. B. 1961. Quantitative studies on tissue transplantation immunity. V. The role of antiserum in enhancement and desensitization. Proc. Roy. Soc., Ser. B. *155*:392-416.

93. Brown, C. A., Draper, P. and Hart, P. D. 1969. Mycobacteria and lysosomes: a paradox. Nature *221*:658-660.

94. Buckingham, S., Heinemann, H. O., Sommers, S. C. and McNary, W. F. 1966. Phospholipid synthesis in the large pulmonary alveolar cell. Amer. J. Path. *48*:1027-1039.

94a. Buechner, H. A. and Ansari, A. 1969. Acute silico-proteinosis. Dis. Chest *55*:274-284.

95. Bullock, W. E. 1968. Studies of immune mechanisms in leprosy. I. Depression of delayed allergic response to skin test antigens. New Eng. J. Med. *278*:298-304.

96. Bullock, W. E., Jr. 1968. Impairment of phytohemagglutinin (PHA) and antigen-induced DNA synthesis in leukocytes cultured from patients with leprosy. (Abstr.) Clin. Res. *16*:328.

97. Bullough, W. S. 1965. Mitotic and functional homeostasis: A speculative review. Cancer Res. *25*:1683-1727.

98. Bullough, W. S. 1967. "The Evolution of Differentiation." Academic Press, London. pp. 94-128.

99. Bullough, W. S. and Laurence, E. B. 1967. Epigenetic mitotic control. *In* "Control of Cellular Growth in Adult Organisms." (Eds. Teir, H. and Rytomaa, T.), Academic Press, London. pp. 28-40.

100. Bullough, W. S., Laurence, E. B., Iversen, O. H. and Elgjo, K. 1967. The vertebrate epidermal chalone. Nature *214*:578-580.

101. Bulmer, D. 1964. The histochemistry of ovarian macrophages in the rat. J. Anat. *98*:313-319.

102. Burch, P. R. J. and Burwell, R. G. 1965. Self and not-self. A clonal induction approach to immunology. Quart. Rev. Biol. *40*:252-279.

103. Burnet, F. M. 1968. Evolution of the immune process in vertebrates. Nature *218*:426-430.
104. Burwell, R. G. 1963. The role of lymphoid tissue in morphostasis. Lancet *ii*:69-74.
105. Byers, S. O. 1960. Lipids and the reticuloendothelial system. Ann. N. Y. Acad. Sci. *88*:240-243.
106. Campbell, D. H. and Garvey, J. S. 1963. Nature of retained antigen and its role in immune mechanisms. Adv. Immunol. *3*:261-313.
107. Canetti, G. 1955. "The Tubercle Bacillus in the Pulmonary Lesion of Man." Springer Publ. Co., New York. pp. 94-97.
108. Cappell, D. F. 1929a. Intravitam and supravital staining. I. The principles and general results. J. Path. Bact. *32*:595-628.
109. Cappell, D. F. 1929b. Intravitam and supravital staining. II. Blood and organs. J. Path. Bact. *32*:629-674.
110. Cappell, D. F. 1929c. Intravitam and supravital staining. III. The nature of the normal lining of the pulmonary alveoli and the origin of the alveolar phagocytes in the light of vital and supravital staining. J. Path. Bact. *32*:675-707.
111. Cappell, D. F. 1930. Intravitam and supravital staining. IV. The cellular reactions following mild irritation of the peritoneum in normal and vitally stained animals with special reference to the origin and nature of the mononuclear cells. J. Path. Bact. *33*:429-452.
112. Carpenter, R. R. and Barsales, P. B. 1967. Uptake by mononuclear phagocytes of protein-coated bentonite particles stabilized with a carbodiimide. J. Immunol. *98*:844-853.
113. Carr, I. 1962. Appositional phagocytosis. J. Path. Bact. *83*:443-448.
114. Carr, I. 1967. The fine structure of cells of the mouse peritoneum. Zeit. für Zellforsch. *80*:534-555.
115. Carr, I., Clegg, E. J. and Meek, G. A. 1968. Sertoli cells as phagocytes: An electron microscopic study. J. Anat. *102*:501-510.
116. Carr, I. and Williams, M. A. 1967. The cellular basis of RE stimulation: The effects on peritoneal cells of stimulation with glyceryl trioleate, studied by EM and autoradiography. Adv. Exp. Med. Biol. *1*:98-107.
117. Carrel, A. 1934. Monocytes as an indicator of certain states of blood serum. Science *80*:565-566.
118. Carrel, A. and Ebeling, A. H. 1926a. Transformation of monocytes into fibroblasts through the action of the Rous virus. J. Exp. Med. *43*:461-468.
119. Carrel, A. and Ebeling, A. H. 1926b. The fundamental properties of the fibroblast and the macrophage. II. The macrophage. J. Exp. Med. *44*:285-305.
120. Carrel, A. and Ingebrigtsen, R. 1912. The production of antibodies by tissues living outside of the organism. J. Exp. Med. *15*:287-291.
121. Carson, M. E. and Dannenberg, A. M., Jr. 1965. Hydrolytic enzymes of rabbit mononuclear exudate cells. II. Lysozyme: Properties and

quantitative assay in tuberculous and control inbred rabbits. J. Immunol. *94*:99-104.

122. Casley-Smith, J. R. and Day, A. J. 1966. The uptake of lipid and lipoprotein by macrophages *in vitro*: an electron microscopical study. Quart. J. Exp. Physiol. *51*:1-10.

123. Chambers, V. C. and Weiser, R. S. 1969. The ultrastructure of target cells and immune macrophages during their interaction *in vitro*. Cancer Res. *29*:301-317.

124. Chandler, J. W., Heise, E. R. and Weiser, R. S. 1969. *In vivo* activities of cytotoxins obtained from cultures of stimulated lymphocytes and macrophages. Proc. Fourth Leukocyte Culture Conference. Appleton-Century-Crofts, New York. (In press.)

125. Chandler, J. W. and Weiser, R. S. 1969. Cellular consequences of aggressor cell-target cell interactions: A review of non-phagocytic mechanisms and cytotoxic mechanisms. (In preparation.)

126. Chang, Y. T. 1964. Long-term cultivation of mouse peritoneal macrophages. J. Natl. Cancer Inst. *32*:19-35.

127. Chapman-Andresen, C. 1962. Studies on pinocytosis in amoebae. Compt. Rend. Trav. Lab. Carlsberg *33*:73-264.

128. Chiller, J. M., Hodgins, H. O., Chambers, V. C. and Weiser, R. S. 1969. Antibody response in rainbow trout (*Salmo gairdneri*). I. Immunocompetent cells in the spleen and anterior kidney. J. Immunol. *102*:1193-1201.

129. Christie, R. V. 1967a. Idiopathic pulmonary hemosiderosis. *In* "Textbook of Medicine," 12th edition. (Eds. Beeson, P. B. and McDermott, W.) W. B. Saunders Co., Philadelphia. pp. 541-542.

130. Christie, R. V. 1967b. Pneumoconiosis. *In* "Textbook of Medicine," 12th edition. (Eds. Beeson, P. B. and McDermott, W.) W. B. Saunders Co., Philadelphia. pp. 529-533.

131. Chrom, S. A. 1935. Studies on the effect of roentgen rays upon the intestinal epithelium and upon the reticulo-endothelial cells of the liver and spleen. Acta Radiol. *16*:641-660.

132. Clark, S. L., Jr. 1963. The thymus in mice of strain 129/J, studied with the electron microscope. Amer. J. Anat. *112*:1-34.

133. Cline, M. J. and Lehrer, R. I. 1968. Phagocytosis by human monocytes. Blood *32*:423-435.

134. Cohen, E. P. and Parks, J. J. 1964. Antibody production by non-immune spleen cells incubated with RNA from immunized mice. Science *144*:1012-1013.

135. Cohn, Z. A. 1964. The fate of bacteria within phagocytic cells. III. Destruction of an *Escherichia coli* agglutinogen within polymorphonuclear leucocytes and macrophages. J. Exp. Med. *120*:869-883.

136. Cohn, Z. A. 1965. The metabolism and physiology of the mononuclear phagocytes. *In* "The Inflammatory Process." (Eds. Zweifach, B. W., Grant, L. and McCluskey, R. T.) Academic Press. New York. pp. 323-353.

137. Cohn, Z. A. 1966. The regulation of pinocytosis in mouse macro-phages. I. Metabolic requirements as defined by the use of in-hibitors. J. Exp. Med. *124*:557-571.

138. Cohn, Z. A. and Benson, B. 1965a. The differentiation of mononuclear phagocytes. Morphology, cytochemistry and biochemistry. J. Exp. Med. *121*:153-170.

139. Cohn, Z. A. and Benson, B. 1965b. The *in vitro* differentiation of mononuclear phagocytes. I. The influence of inhibitors and results of autoradiography. J. Exp. Med. *121*:279-288.

140. Cohn, Z. A. and Benson, B. 1965c. The *in vitro* differentiation of mono-nuclear phagocytes. II. The influence of serum on granule forma-tion, hydrolase production, and pinocytosis. J. Exp. Med. *121*: 835-848.

141. Cohn, Z. A., Fedorko, M. E. and Hirsch, J. G. 1966. The *in vitro* differentiation of mononuclear phagocytes. V. The formation of macrophage lysosomes. J. Exp. Med. *123*:757-766.

142. Cohn, Z. A. and Parks, E. 1967a. The regulation of pinocytosis in mouse macrophages. II. Factors inducing vesicle formation. J. Exp. Med. *125*:213-232.

143. Cohn, Z. A. and Parks, E. 1967b. The regulation of pinocytosis in mouse macrophages. III. The induction of vesicle formation by nucleosides and nucleotides. J. Exp. Med. *125*:457-466.

144. Cohn, Z. A. and Parks, E. 1967c. The regulation of pinocytosis in mouse macrophages. IV. The immunological induction of pino-cytic vesicles, secondary lysosomes, and hydrolytic enzymes. J. Exp. Med. *125*:1091-1104.

145. Cohn, Z. A. and Weiner, E. 1963. The particulate hydrolases of macro-phages. I. Comparative enzymology, isolation and properties. J. Exp. Med. *118*:991-1008.

146. Colwell, C. A., Hess, A. R. and Tavaststjerna, M. 1963. Mononuclear cells from animals of divergent susceptibility to tuberculosis. Amer. Rev. Resp. Dis. *88*:37-46.

147. Comolli, R. 1967. Cytotoxicity of silica and liberation of lysosomal enzymes. J. Path. Bact. *93*:241-253.

148. Cooper, G. N. 1964. Functional modification of reticuloendothelial cells by simple triglycerides. J. Reticuloendothel. Soc. *1*:50-67.

149. Cooper, G. N. and West, D. 1962. Effects of simple lipids on the phagocytic properties of peritoneal macrophages. I. Stimulatory effects of glyceryl trioleate. Aust. J. Exp. Biol. Med. Sci. *40*: 485-498.

150. Coppel, S. and Youmans, G. P. 1969. Specificity of the anamnestic response produced by *Listeria monocytogenes* or *Mycobacterium tuberculosis* to challenge with *Listeria monocytogenes*. J. Bact. *97*:127-133.

151. Cox, A. W., Schroeder, N. F. and Ristic, M. 1965. Erythrophagocytosis associated with anemia in rats infected with *Plasmodium berghei*. J. Parasit. *51*:35-36.

152. Croft, J. D., Jr., Swisher, S. N., Jr., Gilliland, B. C., Bakemeier, R. F., Leddy, J. P. and Weed, R. I. 1968. Coombs'-test positivity induced by drugs. Ann. Intern. Med. *68*:176-187.

153. Crome, P. and Mollison, P. L. 1964. Splenic destruction of Rh-sensitized and of heated red cells. Brit. J. Haematol. *10*:137-154.

154. Curran, R. C. and Rowsell, E. V. 1958. The application of the diffusion-chamber technique to the study of silicosis. J. Path. Bact. *76*:561-568.

155. Dacie, J. V. 1960. "The Hemolytic Anaemias. Congenital and Acquired. Part I. The Congenital Anaemias." Grune & Stratton, Inc., New York. pp. 3-6.

156. Daland, G. A., Gottlieb, L., Wallerstein, R. O. and Castle, W. B. 1956. Hematologic observations in bacterial endocarditis: especially the prevalence of histiocytes and the elevation and variation of the white cell count in blood from the ear lobe. J. Lab. Clin. Med. *48*:827-845.

157. Dannenberg, A. M., Jr. 1968. Cellular hypersensitivity and cellular immunity in the pathogenesis of tuberculosis: Specificity, systemic and local nature, and associated macrophage enzymes. Bact. Rev. *32*:85-102.

158. Dannenberg, A. M., Jr. and Bennett, W. E. 1964. Hydrolytic enzymes of rabbit mononuclear exudate cells. I. Quantitative assay and properties of certain proteases, non-specific esterases, and lipases of mononuclear and polymorphonuclear cells and erythrocytes. J. Cell Biol. *21*:1-13.

159. Dannenberg, A. M., Jr., Burstone, M. S., Walter, P. C. and Kinsley, J. W. 1963. A histochemical study of phagocytic and enzymatic functions of rabbit mononuclear and polymorphonuclear exudate cells and alveolar macrophages. I. Survey and quantitation of enzymes, and states of cellular activation. J. Cell Biol. *17*:465-486.

160. Dannenberg, A. M., Jr., Meyer, O. T., Esterly, J. R. and Kambara, T. 1968. The local nature of immunity in tuberculosis, illustrated histochemically in dermal BCG lesions. J. Immunol. *100*:931-941.

161. Dannenberg, A. M., Jr., Walter, P. C. and Kapral, F. A. 1963. A histochemical study of phagocytic and enzymatic functions of rabbit mononuclear and polymorphonuclear exudate cells and alveolar macrophages. II. The effect of particle ingestion on enzyme activity; two phases of *in vitro* activation. J. Immunol. *90*:448-465.

162. Dargeon, H. W. K. 1966. "Reticuloendothelioses in Childhood. A Clinical Survey." Charles C Thomas, Springfield, Ill. 127 pp.

163. Davey, M. J. and Asherson, G. L. 1967. Cytophilic antibody. I. Nature of the macrophage receptor. Immunology *12*:13-20.

164. David, J. R. 1966. Delayed hypersensitivity *in vitro*: Its mediation by cell-free substances formed by lymphoid cell-antigen interraction. Proc. Nat. Acad. Sci. *56*:72-77.

165. David, J. R. 1968a. Studies on the mechanisms of delayed hypersensitivity. Intern. Symp. Immunopath. *5*:253-262.

166. David, J. R. 1968b. Macrophage migration. Fed. Proc. *27*:6-12.

167. David, J. R., Al-Askari, S., Lawrence, H. S. and Thomas, L. 1964a. Delayed hypersensitivity *in vitro*. I. The specificity of inhibition of cell migration by antigens. J. Immunol. *93*:264-273.

168. David, J. R., Lawrence, H. S. and Thomas, L. 1964b. Delayed hypersensitivity *in vitro*. II. Effect of sensitive cells on normal cells in the presence of antigen. J. Immunol. *93*:274-278.

169. David, J. R., Lawrence, H. S. and Thomas, L. 1964c. Delayed hypersensitivity *in vitro*. III. The specificity of hapten-protein conjugates in the inhibition of cell migration. J. Immunol. *93*:279-282.

170. David, J. R., Lawrence, H. S. and Thomas, L. 1964d. The *in vitro* desensitization of sensitive cells by trypsin. J. Exp. Med. *120*:1189-1200.

171. Day, A. J. 1960a. Cholesterol esterase activity of rabbit macrophages. Quart. J. Exp. Physiol. *45*:55-59.

172. Day, A. J. 1960b. Removal of cholesterol from reticulo-endothelial cells. Brit. J. Exp. Path. *41*:112-118.

173. Day, A. J. 1960c. Oxidation of ^{14}C-labelled chylomicron fat and ^{14}C-labelled unesterified fatty acids by macrophages *in vitro* and the effect of clearing factor. Quart. J. Exp. Physiol. *45*:220-228.

174. Day, A. J. 1961. A comparison of the oxidation of cholesterol-26-^{14}C, palmitate-1-^{14}C and tripalmitin-1-^{14}C by macrophages *in vitro*. Quart. J. Exp. Physiol. *46*:383-388.

175. Day, A. J. 1967. Lipid metabolism by macrophages and its relation to atherosclerosis. Adv. Lipid Res. *5*:185-207.

176. Day, A. J. and Fidge, N. H. 1964. Incorporation of C^{14}-labeled acetate into lipids by macrophages *in vitro*. J. Lipid Res. *5*:163-168.

177. Day, A. J., Fidge, N. H., Gould-Hurst, P. R. S. and Wilkinson, G. K. 1965. Metabolism of cholesterol ester by reticulo-endothelial cells. Quart. J. Exp. Physiol. *50*:248-255.

178. Day, A. J., Fidge, N. H., Gould-Hurst, P. R. S., Wahlqvist, M. L. and Wilkinson, G. K. 1966. Uptake and metabolism of ^{14}C-labelled triglyceride by reticulo-endothelial cells. Quart. J. Exp. Physiol. *51*:11-17.

179. Day, A. J. and French, J. E. 1959. The synthesis and hydrolysis of cholesteryl ester by cells of the reticulo-endothelial system. Quart. J. Exp. Physiol. *44*:239-243.

180. Day, A. J. and Gould-Hurst, P. R. S. 1963. The effect of lecithin on cholesterol esterase activity of rabbit macrophages. Aust. J. Exp. Biol. Med. Sci. *41*:323-330.

181. Day, A. J., Gould-Hurst, P. R. S., Steinborner, R. and Wahlqvist, M. L. 1965. Removal of double-labelled lipid mixtures and double-labelled lipoprotein preparations by reticulo-endothelial cells. J. Atheroscler. Res. *5*:466-473.

182. Dempster, W. J., Harrison, C. V. and Shackman, R. 1964. Rejection processes in human homotransplanted kidney. Brit. Med. J. 2:969-976.
183. Deno, R. A. 1937. Uterine macrophages in the mouse and their relation to involution. Amer. J. Anat. 60:433-471.
184. Deodhar, S. D. and Bhagwat, A. G. 1967. Desquamative interstitial pneumonia-like syndrome in rabbits, produced experimentally by Freund's adjuvant. Arch. Path. 84:54-58.
185. Dharmendra and Chatterjee, K. R. 1955. Prognostic value of the lepromin test in contacts of leprosy cases. Leprosy Ind. 27:149.
186. DiCarlo, F. J., Haynes, L. J., Coutinho, C. B. and Phillips, G. E. 1965. Pentobarbital sleeping time and RES stimulation. J. Reticuloendothel. Soc. 2:367-378.
187. Dienes, L. 1932. Factors conditioning the development of the tuberculin type of hypersensitivity. J. Immunol. 23:11-27.
188. Dierks, R. E. and Shepard, C. C. 1968. Effect of phytohemagglutinin and various mycobacterial antigens on lymphocyte cultures from leprosy patients. Proc. Soc. Exp. Biol. Med. 127:391-395.
189. DiLuzio, N. R. 1955. Effects of x-irradiation and choline on the reticulo-endothelial system of the rat. Amer. J. Physiol. 181:595-598.
190. Dineen, J. K. and Wagland, B. M. 1966. The cellular transfer of immunity to Trichostrongylus colubriformis in an isogenic strain of guinea pig. II. The relative susceptibility of the larvae and adult stages of the parasite to immunological attack. Immunology 11:47-57.
191. Dineen, J. K., Wagland, B. M. and Ronai, P. M. 1968. The cellular transfer of immunity to Trichostrongylus colubriformis in an isogenic strain of guinea pig. III. The localization and functional activity of immune lymph node cells following syngeneic and allogeneic transfer. Immunology 15:335-341.
192. Dixon, F. J., Bukantz, S. C., Dammin, G. J. and Talmage, D. W. 1953. Fate of I131-labeled bovine gamma globulin in rabbits. In "The Nature and Significance of the Antibody Response." (Ed. Pappenheimer, A. M., Jr.) Columbia Univ. Press, New York. pp. 170-182.
193. Doan, C. A. and Sabin, F. R. 1926. Normal and pathological fragmentation of red blood cells; The phagocytosis of these fragments by desquamated endothelial cells of the blood stream; The correlation of the peroxidase reaction with phagocytosis in mononuclear cells. J. Exp. Med. 43:839-850.
194. Dobson, E. L., Kelly, L. S. and Finney, C. R. 1967. Kinetics of the phagocytosis of repeated injections of colloidal carbon: Blockade, a latent period or stimulation? A question of timing and dose. Adv. Exp. Med. Biol. 1:63-73.
195. Donaldson, D. M., Marcus, S., Gyi, K. K. and Perkins, E. H. 1956. The influence of immunization and total body x-irradiation on intracellular digestion by peritoneal phagocytes. J. Immunol. 76:192-199.

196. Dumonde, D. C. 1967a. The role of the macrophage in delayed hypersensitivity. Brit. Med. Bull. *23*:9-14.

197. Dumonde, D. C. 1967b. The role of the macrophage in transplantation immunity. (Sympos. Tissue Org. Transplant.) Suppl., J. Clin. Path. *20*:430-436.

198. Dumonde, D. C., Howson, W. T. and Wolstencroft, R. A. 1968. The role of macrophages and lymphocytes in reactions of delayed hypersensitivity. Intern. Symp. Immunopath. *5*:263-278.

199. Dumont, A. and Sheldon, H. 1965. Changes in the fine structure of macrophages in experimentally produced tuberculous granulomas in hamsters. Lab. Invest. *14*:2034-2055.

200. Dunn, W. B., Hardin, J. H. and Spicer, S. S. 1968. Ultrastructural localization of myeloperoxidase in human neutrophil and rabbit heterophil and eosinophil leukocytes. Blood *32*:935-944.

201. Dutton, R. W. 1967. *In vitro* studies of immunological responses of lymphoid cells. Adv. Immunol. *6*:253-336.

202. Ebert, R. H. and Florey, H. W. 1939. The extravascular development of the monocyte observed *in vivo*. Brit. J. Exp. Path. *20*:342-356.

203. Ebert, R. V. 1967. Diffuse interstitial pulmonary fibrosis. *In* "Textbook of Medicine," 12th edition. (Eds. Beeson, P. B. and McDermott, W.) W. B. Saunders Co., Philadelphia. pp. 514-515.

204. Ehrenreich, B. A. and Cohn, Z. A. 1968a. Pinocytosis by macrophages. J. Reticuloendothel. Soc. *5*:230-242.

205. Ehrenreich, B. A. and Cohn, Z. A. 1968b. Fate of hemoglobin pinocytosed by macrophages *in vitro*. J. Cell Biol. *38*:244-248.

206. Elberg, S. S. 1960. Cellular immunity. Bact. Rev. *24*:67-95.

207. Elsbach, P. 1965. Uptake of fat by phagocytic cells. An examination of the role of phagocytosis. II. Rabbit alveolar macrophages. Biochim. Biophys. Acta *98*:420-431.

208. Elsbach, P. 1968. Increased synthesis of phospholipid during phagocytosis. J. Clin. Invest. *47*:2217-2229.

209. Elves, M. W. 1966. "The Lymphocytes." Lloyd-Luke Ltd., London. p. 120.

210. Elves, M. W. 1967. The effect of polymorphonuclear leukocytes on blast transformation of lymphocytes in human mixed leukocyte cultures. Transplantation *5*:1416-1422.

211. Epstein, W. L. and Krasnobrod, H. 1968. The origin of epithelioid cells in experimental granulomas of man. Lab. Invest. *18*:190-195.

212. Essner, E. 1960. An electron microscopic study of erythrophagocytosis. J. Biophys. and Biochem. Cytol. *7*:329-333.

213. Everett, N. B. and Tyler (Caffrey), R. W. 1967. Lymphopoiesis in the thymus and other tissues: Functional implications. Intern. Rev. Cytol. *22*:205-237.

214. Fagraeus, A. 1948. The plasma cellular reaction and its relation to the formation of antibodies *in vitro*. J. Immunol. *58*:1-13.

215. Fauve, R. M. and Dekaris, D. 1968. Macrophage spreading: Inhibition in delayed hypersensitivity. Science *160*:795-796.

216. Fedorko, M. E., Hirsch, J. G. and Cohn, Z. A. 1968. Autophagic vacuoles produced *in vitro*. I. Studies on cultured macrophages exposed to chloroquine. J. Cell Biol. *38*:377-391.

217. Feldman, M. and Bleiberg, I. 1967. Studies on the feedback regulation of haemopoiesis. *In* "Cell Differentiation." (Eds. De Reuck, A. V. S. and Knight, J.) Ciba Fndn. Symposium. Little, Brown & Co., Boston. pp. 79-89.

218. Feldman, M. and Gallily, R. 1967. Cell interactions in the induction of antibody formation. Cold Spring Harbor Symp. Quant. Biol. *32*:415-421.

219. Felix, M. D. and Dalton, A. J. 1955. A phase-contrast microscope study of free cells native to the peritoneal fluid of DBA/2 mice. J. Nat. Cancer Inst. *16*:415-445.

220. Felton, L. D. 1949. The significance of antigen in animal tissues. J. Immunol. *61*:107-117.

221. Fernex, M. 1968. "The Mast-Cell System. Its Relationship to Atherosclerosis, Fibrosis and Eosinophils." Williams & Wilkins Co., Baltimore. p. 88.

222. Fisher, B. and Fisher, E. R. 1964. Tissue transplantation and the reticuloendothelial system. I. Effect of skin grafts in normal animals. Transplantation *2*:228-234.

223. Fishman, M. 1959. Antibody formation in tissue culture. Nature *183*: 1200-1201.

224. Fishman, M. 1961. Antibody formation *in vitro*. J. Exp. Med. *114*: 837-856.

225. Fishman, M. and Adler, F. L. 1963. Antibody formation initiated *in vitro*. II. Antibody synthesis in X-irradiated recipients of diffusion chambers containing nucleic acid derived from macrophages incubated with antigen. J. Exp. Med. *117*:595-602.

226. Fishman, M. and Adler, F. L. 1967. The role of macrophage-RNA in the immune response. Cold Spring Harbor Symp. Quant. Biol. *32*:343-347.

227. Fitzgeorge, R. B., Solotorovsky, M. and Smith, H. 1967. The behavior of *Brucella abortus* within macrophages separated from the blood of normal and immune cattle by adherence to glass. Brit. J. Exp. Path. *48*:522-528.

228. Flemming, K. B. P. 1967. Pharmacological stimulation and depression of the phagocytic function of the RES. Adv. Exp. Med. Biol. *1*:188-196.

229. Fletcher, J. and Huehns, E. R. 1968. Function of transferrin. Nature *218*:1211-1214.

230. Florey, H. 1962. "General Pathology." W. B. Saunders Co., Philadelphia. p. 129.

231. Foley, E. J. 1953. Antigenic properties of methylcholanthrene-induced tumors in mice of the strain of origin. Cancer Res. *13*:835-837.

232. Fong, J., Schneider, P. and Elberg, S. S. 1956. Studies on tubercle bacillus-monocyte relationship. I. Quantitative analysis of effect of

serum of animals vaccinated with B.C.G. upon bacterium-monocyte system. J. Exp. Med. *104*:455-465.

233. Fong, J., Schneider, P. and Elberg, S. S. 1957. Studies on tubercle bacillus-monocyte relationship. II. Induction of monocyte degeneration by bacteria and culture filtrate: Specificity of serum and monocyte effects on resistance to degeneration. J. Exp. Med. *105*:25-37.

234. Forbes, I. J. 1965. Induction of mitosis in macrophages by endotoxin. J. Immunol. *94*:37-39.

235. Forbes, I. J. 1966. Mitosis in mouse peritoneal macrophages. J. Immunol. *96*:734-743.

236. Forbes, I. J. and Mackaness, G. B. 1963. Mitosis in macrophages. Lancet *ii*:1203-1204.

237. Ford, C. E., Micklem, H. S. and Ogden, D. A. 1968. Evidence for the existence of a lymphoid stem cell. Lancet *i*:621-622.

238. Forteza, G. 1964. "Atlas of Blood Cytology, Cytomorphology, Cytochemistry and Cytogenetics." Grune & Stratton, New York. 511 pp.

239. Franzl, R. E. and McMaster, P. D. 1968a. The primary immune response in mice. I. The enhancement and suppression of hemolysin production by a bacterial endotoxin. J. Exp. Med. *127*:1087-1107.

240. Franzl, R. E. and McMaster, P. D. 1968b. The primary immune response in mice. II. Cellular responses of lymphoid tissue accompanying the enhancement or complete suppression of antibody formation by a bacterial endotoxin. J. Exp. Med. *127*:1109-1125.

241. Fred, R. K. and Shore, M. L. 1967. Application of a mathematical model to the study of RES phagocytosis in mice. Adv. Exp. Med. Biol. *1*:1-17.

242. Freedman, H. H. 1960. Reticuloendothelial system and passive transfer of endotoxin tolerance. Ann. N. Y. Acad. Sci. *88*:99-106.

243. Frei, P. C., Benacerraf, B. and Thorbecke, G. J. 1965. Phagocytosis of the antigen, a crucial step in the induction of the immune response. Proc. Nat. Acad. Sci. *53*:20-23.

244. Fresen, O. 1960. The concept and importance of the reticuloendothelial system considered from the morphological aspect. *In* "Reticuloendothelial Structure and Function." (Ed. Heller, J. H.) Ronald Press Co., New York. pp. 3-21.

245. Frey, J. R. and Wenk, P. 1957. Experimental studies on the pathogenesis of contact eczema in the guinea-pig. Int. Arch. Allergy *11*:81-100.

246. French, J. E. and Morris, B. 1960. The uptake and storage of lipid particles in lymph-glands in the rat. J. Path. Bact. *79*:11-19.

247. Friedman, H. 1964. Antibody plaque formation by normal spleen cell cultures exposed *in vitro* to RNA from immune mice. Science *146*:934-936.

248. Frolova, M. A. and Sokolova, E. I. 1964. Tissue culture as a method for study of cellular reactivity in antitoxic immunity. Fed. Proc. (Transl. Suppl.) *23*:1340-1342.

249. Furness, G. and Axelrod, A. E. 1959. The effect of deficiencies of thiamine, pyridoxine and pantothenic acid on the macrophages of the rat. J. Immunol. *83*:133-137.

250. Furth, R. van and Cohn, Z. A. 1968. The origin and kinetics of mononuclear phagocytes. J. Exp. Med. *128*:415-435.

251. Gabrieli, E. R. and Auskaps, A. A. 1953. The effect of whole body x-irradiation on the reticulo-endothelial system as demonstrated by the use of radioactive chromium phosphate. Yale J. Biol. Med. *26*:159-169.

252. Gall, E. A. 1958. The cytological identity and interrelationship of mesenchymal cells of lymphoid tissue. Ann. N. Y. Acad. Sci. *73*:120-130.

253. Gallily, R. and Feldman, M. 1966. The induction of antibody production in x-irradiated animals by macrophages that interacted with antigen. Israel J. Med. Sci. *2*:358-361.

254. Gallily, R. and Feldman, M. 1967a. The role of macrophages in the induction of antibody in x-irradiated animals. Immunology *12*: 197-206.

255. Gallily, R. and Feldman, M. 1967b. The cellular components in the induction of antibody by x-irradiated animals. *In* "Germinal Centers in Immune Responses." (Eds. Cottier, H., Odartchenko, N., Schindler, R. and Congdon, C. C.) Springer-Verlag, New York. pp. 333-336.

256. Garvey, J. S. 1961. Separation and *in vitro* culture of cells from liver tissue. Nature *191*:972-974.

257. Garvey, J. S. and Campbell, D. H. 1957. The retention of S^{35}-labeled bovine serum albumin in normal and immunized rabbit liver tissue. J. Exp. Med. *105*:361-372.

258. Gell, P. G. H. and Hinde, I. T. 1953. The effect of cortisone on macrophage activity in mice. Brit. J. Exp. Path. *34*:273-275.

259. George, M. and Vaughan, J. H. 1962. *In vitro* cell migration as a model for delayed hypersensitivity. Proc. Soc. Exp. Biol. Med. *111*:514-521.

260. Gershon, R. K., Carter, R. L. and Lane, N. J. 1967. Studies on homotransplantable lymphomas in hamsters. IV. Observations on macrophages in the expression of tumor immunity. Amer. J. Path. *51*: 1111-1133.

261. Gershon, H. and Feldman, M. 1968. Studies on the immune reconstitution of sublethally irradiated mice by peritoneal macrophages. Immunology *15*:827-835.

262. Ghiringhelli, L. and Pernis, B. 1958. Augmento della produzione di anticorpi nei conigli trattati con tridimite per via endovenosa. Med. Lavoro *49*:665-671.

263. Gill, F. A. and Cole, R. M. 1965. The fate of a bacterial antigen (streptococcal M protein) after phagocytosis by macrophages. J. Immunol. *94*:898-915.

264. Gill, F. A., Kaye, D. and Hook, E. W. 1966. The influence of erythro-

phagocytosis on the interaction of macrophages and salmonella *in vitro*. J. Exp. Med. *124*:173-183.

265. Gillman, J., Gillman, T. and Gilbert, C. 1949. Reticulosis and reticulum-cell tumours of the liver produced in rats by Trypan blue with reference to hepatic necrosis and fibrosis. S. Afr. J. Med. Sci. *14*: 21-84.

266. Gillman, T. and Wright, L. J. 1966. Autoradiographic evidence suggesting *in vivo* transformation of some blood mononuclears in repair and fibrosis. Nature *209*:1086-1090.

267. Gilman, R. and Trowell, O. A. 1965. The effect of radiation on the activity of reticuloendothelial cells in organ cultures of lymph node and thymus. Intern. J. Rad. Biol. *9*:313-322.

268. Globerson, A. and Auerbach, R. 1965. Primary immune reactions in organ cultures. Science *149*:991-993.

269. Goldfischer, S., Kikkawa, Y. and Hoffman, L. 1968. The demonstration of acid hydrolase activities in the inclusion bodies of Type II alveolar cells and other lysosomes in the rabbit lung. J. Histochem. Cytochem. *16*:102-109.

270. Goldstein, E. and Green, G. M. 1966. The effect of acute renal failure on the bacterial clearance mechanisms of the lung. J. Lab. Clin. Med. *68*:531-542.

271. Goodman, J. W. 1964. On the origin of peritoneal fluid cells. Blood *23*:18-26.

272. Gordon, A. S. and Katsh, G. F. 1949. The relation of the adrenal cortex to the structure and phagocytic activity of the macrophagic system. Ann. N. Y. Acad. Sci. *52*:1-30.

273. Gordon, J. 1968. Role of monocytes in the mixed leukocyte culture reaction. Proc. Soc. Exp. Biol. Med. *127*:30-33.

274. Gordon, L. E., Cooper, D. B. and Miller, C. P. 1955. Clearance of bacteria from the blood of irradiated rabbits. Proc. Soc. Exp. Biol. Med. *89*:577-579.

275. Gorer, P. A. 1958. Some reactions of H-2 antibodies *in vitro* and *in vivo*. Ann. N. Y. Acad. Sci. *73*:707-721.

276. Gottlieb, A. A. 1968. Antigens, RNAs, and macrophages. J. Reticuloendothel. Soc. *5*:270-281.

277. Gottlieb, A. A., Glišin, V. R. and Doty, P. 1967. Studies on macrophage RNA involved in antibody production. Proc. Nat. Acad. Sci. *57*:1849-1856.

278. Gough, J. and Elves, M. W. 1966. Studies of lymphocytes and their derivative cells *in vitro*. I. Biochemical constituents. Acta Haemat. (Basel) *36*:344-349.

279. Gough, J. and Elves, M. W. 1967. Studies of lymphocytes and their derivative cells *in vitro*. II. Enzyme cytochemistry. Acta Haemat. (Basel) *37*:42-52.

280. Gough, J., Elves, M. W. and Israëls, M. C. G. 1965. The formation of macrophages from lymphocytes *in vitro*. Exp. Cell Res. *38*:476-482.

281. Gowans, J. L. and McGregor, D. D. 1965. The immunological activities of lymphocytes. Progr. Allergy 9:1-78.
282. Gowland, E. 1968. The physico-chemical properties of cytophilic antibody. Aust. J. Exp. Biol. Med. Sci. 46:73-81.
283. Granger, G. A. and Weiser, R. S. 1964. Homograft target cells: Specific destruction in vitro by contact interaction with immune macrophages. Science 145:1427-1429.
284. Granger, G. A. and Weiser, R. S. 1966. Homograft target cells: Contact destruction in vitro by immune macrophages. Science 151: 97-99.
285. Granger, G. A. and Williams, T. W. 1968. Lymphocyte cytotoxicity in vitro: Activation and release of a cytotoxic factor. Nature 218:1253-1254.
286. Green, G. M. and Carolin, D. 1967. The depressant effect of cigarette smoke on the in vitro antibacterial activity of alveolar macrophages. New Eng. J. Med. 276:421-427.
287. Green, G. M. and Kass, E. H. 1964. The role of the alveolar macrophage in the clearance of bacteria from the lung. J. Exp. Med. 119:167-176.
288. Greenberg, M. S. 1964. Ear lobe histiocytosis as a clue to the diagnosis of subacute bacterial endocarditis. Ann. Intern. Med. 61:124-127.
289. Grogg, E. and Pearse, A. G. E. 1952. The enzymic and lipid histochemistry of experimental tuberculosis. Brit. J. Exp. Path. 33: 567-576.
290. Gurdon, J. B. and Uehlinger, V. 1966. "Fertile" intestine nuclei. Nature 210:1240-1241.
291. Hadler, W. A., Ferreira, A. L. and Ziti, L. M. 1965. An attempt to stimulate and depress the functional activity of the inflammatory cells from lesions experimentally induced by M. leprae and M. lepraemurium. Leprosy Rev. 36:163-170.
292. Hahn, H. H., Char, D. C., Postel, W. B. and Wood, W. B., Jr. 1967. Studies on the pathogenesis of fever: XV. Production of endogenous pyrogen by peritoneal macrophages. J. Exp. Med. 126:385-394.
293. Hall, J. G. and Morris, B. 1965. The origin of the cells in the efferent lymph from a single lymph node. J. Exp. Med. 121:901-910.
294. Halpern, B. N., Biozzi, G. and Stiffel, C. 1963. Action de l'extrait microbien Wxb 3148 sur l'évolution des tumeurs éxperimentales. Colloques internationaux du C.N.R.S. 115:221-236.
295. Han, S. H. 1966. Studies on tuberculin sensitivity. Ph.D. thesis. University of Washington. Seattle, Washington.
296. Hancox, N. M. 1949. The osteoclast. Biol. Rev. 24:448-471.
297. Harington, J. S. 1963. Some biological actions of silica: Their part in the pathogenesis of silicosis. S. Afr. Med. J. 37:451-456.
298. Harris, G. 1967. Macrophages from tolerant rabbits as mediators of a specific immunological response in vitro. Immunology 12:159-163.
299. Harris, H. 1953. Chemotaxis of monocytes. Brit. J. Exp. Path. 34: 276-279.

300. Harris, H. 1954. Role of chemotaxis in inflammation. Physiol. Rev. *34*:529-562.
301. Harris, H. 1966. Hybrid cells from mouse and man: a study in genetic regulation. Proc. Roy. Soc., Ser. B *166*:358-368.
302. Harris, H. and Barclay, W. R. 1955. A method for measuring the respiration of animal cells *in vitro*, with some observations on the macrophages of the rabbit. Brit. J. Exp. Path. *36*:592-598.
303. Harris, H. R. 1958. Foam cells in the stroma of carcinoma of the body of the uterus and uterine cervical polypi. J. Clin. Path. *11*:19-22.
304. Hatch, T. F. and Kindsvatter, V. H. 1947. Lung retention of quartz dust smaller than one-half micron. J. Industr. Hyg. and Toxicol. *29*:342-346.
305. Heilman, D. H. 1963. Tissue culture methods for studying delayed allergy: A review. Texas Rept. Biol. Med. *21*:136-157.
306. Heilman, D. H. 1964. Cellular aspects of the action of endotoxin: The role of the macrophage. *In* "Bacterial Endotoxins." (Eds. Landy, M. and Braun, W.) Rutgers Intern. Symp. Quinn and Boden Co., Inc., Rahway, N. J. pp. 610-617.
307. Heilman, D. H. 1965. The selective toxicity of endotoxin for phagocytic cells of the reticuloendothelial system. Int. Arch. Allerg. *26*:63-79.
308. Heinmets, F. 1968. Cell-cell interaction. Currents in Mod. Biol. *1*: 299-313.
309. Heise, E. R., Han, S. and Weiser, R. S. 1968. *In vitro* studies on the mechanism of macrophage migration inhibition in tuberculin sensitivity. J. Immunol. *101*:1004-1015.
310. Heise, E. R., Myrvik, Q. N. and Leake, E. S. 1965. Effect of bacillus Calmette-Guérin on the levels of acid phosphatase, lysozyme and cathepsin in rabbit alveolar macrophages. J. Immunol. *95*:125-130.
311. Heise, E. R. and Weiser, R. S. 1969. Tuberculin sensitivity: Relation of cytotoxin to local cutaneous and systemic reactions. (In preparation.)
312. Heller, J. H. 1958. Measurement of the function of the reticuloendothelium. Ann. N. Y. Acad. Sci. *73*:212-220.
313. Heller, J. H. 1960. Nontoxic RES stimulatory lipids. Ann. N. Y. Acad. Sci. *88*:116-121.
314. Heller, J. H., Ransom, J. P. and Pasternak, V. Z. 1963. New advances in the stimulation of the R.E.S. Colloques internationaux du C.N.R.S. *115*:89-105.
315. Hellström, K. E. and Hellström, I. 1969. Cellular immunity against tumor antigens. Adv. Cancer Res. *12*:167-223.
316. Hellström, K. E. and Möller, G. 1965. Immunological and immunogenetic aspects of tumor transplantation. Progr. Allergy *9*:158-245.
317. Helminen, H. J. and Ericsson, J. L. E. 1968a. Studies on mammary gland involution. I. On the ultrastructure of the lactating mammary gland. J. Ultrastruct. Res. *25*:193-213.

318. Helminen, H. J. and Ericsson, J. L. E. 1968b. Studies on mammary gland involution. II. Ultrastructural evidence for auto- and hetero-phagocytosis. J. Ultrastruct. Res. *25*:214-227.

319. Helminen, H. J. and Ericsson, J. L. E. 1968c. Studies on mammary gland involution. III. Alterations outside auto- and heterophagocytic pathways for cytoplasmic degradation. J. Ultrastruct. Res. *25*:228-239.

320. Helminen, H. J., Ericsson, J. L. E. and Orrenius, S. 1968. Studies on mammary gland involution. IV. Histochemical and biochemical observations on alterations in lysosomes and lysosomal enzymes. J. Ultrastruct. Res. *25*:240-252.

321. Heppleston, A. G. 1963. The disposal of inhaled particulate matter: A unifying hyphothesis. Amer. J. Path. *42*:119-135.

322. Heppleston, A. G. and Styles, J. A. 1967. Activity of a macrophage factor in collagen formation by silica. Nature *214*:521-522.

323. Hersh, E. M. and Harris, J. E. 1968. Macrophage-lymphocyte inter-action in the antigen-induced blastogenic response of human periph-eral blood leukocytes. J. Immunol. *100*:1184-1194.

324. Hetherington, D. C. and Pierce, E. J. 1931. The transformation of monocytes into macrophages and epithelioid cells in tissue cultures of buffy coat. Arch. Exp. Zellforsch. *12*:1-10.

324a. Holder, I. A. and Sword, C. P. 1969. Characterization and biological activity of the monocytosis-producing agent of *Listeria mono-cytogenes*. J. Bact. *97*:603-611.

325. Holland, J. J. and Pickett, M. J. 1958. A cellular basis of immunity in experimental *Brucella* infection. J. Exp. Med. *108*:343-360.

326. Holmes, B., Page, A. R. and Good, R. A. 1967. Studies of the meta-bolic activity of leukocytes from patients with a genetic abnor-mality of phagocytic function. J. Clin. Invest. *46*:1422-1432.

327. Holter, H. 1959a. Problems of pinocytosis, with special regard to amoebae. Ann. N. Y. Acad. Sci. *78*:524-537.

328. Holter, H. 1959b. Pinocytosis. Int. Rev. Cytol. *8*:481-504.

329. Holtzer, J. D. 1967. Experimental delayed type allergy without demon-strable antibodies. II. *In vitro* activity of reticulo-endothelial cells. Immunology *12*:713-723.

330. Holtzer, J. D. and Winkler, K. C. 1967. Experimental delayed type allergy without demonstrable antibodies. I. Absence of cytophilic antibodies. Immunology *12*:701-712.

330a. Holub, M. and Hauser, R. E. 1969. Lung alveolar histiocytes engaged in antibody production. Immunology *17*:207-226.

331. Honjin, R. 1963. Electron microscopic studies on the neuroglial cells and the vascular bed of the central nervous system. *In* "Mor-phology of Neuroglia." (Ed. Nakai, J.) Charles C Thomas, Springfield, Ill. pp. 53-64.

332. Hosokawa, H. and Mannen, H. 1963. Some aspects of the histology of neuroglia. *In* "Morphology of Neuroglia." (Ed. Nakai, J.) Charles C Thomas, Springfield, Ill. pp 1-52.

333. Howard, J. G. 1964. Stimulation of the Kupffer cells during graft-versus-host reaction in the mouse: Its use, significance and modification. Abstract. RES: J. Reticuloendothel. Soc. *1*:360.

334. Howard, J. G. and Benacerraf, B. 1966. Properties of macrophage receptors for cytophilic antibodies. Brit. J. Exp. Path. *47*:193-200.

335. Howard, J. G., Boak, J. L. and Christie, G. H. 1966. Further studies on the transformation of thoracic duct cells into liver macrophages. Ann. N. Y. Acad. Sci. *129*:327-339.

336. Howard, J. G. and Wardlaw, A. C. 1958. The opsonic effect of normal serum on the uptake of bacteria by the reticulo-endothelial system. Immunology *1*:338-352.

337. Hsu, H. S. 1965. *In vitro* studies on the interactions between macrophages of rabbits and tubercle bacilli. II. Cellular and humoral aspects of acquired resistance. Amer. Rev. Resp. Dis. *91*:499-509.

338. Hsu, H. S. and Kapral, F. A. 1960. The suppressed multiplication of tubercle bacilli within macrophages derived from triiodothyronine-treated guinea pigs. Amer. Rev. Resp. Dis. *81*:881-887.

339. Huber, J. and Fudenberg, H. H. 1968. Receptor sites of human monocytes for IgG. Int. Arch. Allergy *34*:18-31.

340. Huber, H., Polley, M. J., Linscott, W. D., Fudenberg, H. H. and Müller-Eberhard, H. J. 1968. Human monocytes: Distinct receptor sites for the third component of complement and for Immunoglobulin G. Science *162*:1281-1283.

341. Humphrey, J. H. 1967. Cell-mediated immunity—general perspectives. Brit. Med. Bull. *23*:93-97.

342. Hunt, W. B., Jr. and Myrvik, Q. N. 1964. Demonstration of antibody in rabbit alveolar macrophages with failure to transfer antibody production. J. Immunol. *93*:677-681.

343. Hurd, E. R. and Ziff, M. 1968. Studies on the anti-inflammatory action of 6-mercaptopurine. J. Exp. Med. *128*:785-800.

344. Ichikawa, Y., Pluznik, D. H. and Sachs, L. 1966. *In vitro* control of the development of macrophage and granulocyte colonies. Proc. Nat. Acad. Sci. *56*:488-495.

345. Ichikawa, Y., Pluznik, D. H. and Sachs, L. 1967. Feedback inhibition of the development of macrophage and granulocyte colonies. I. Inhibition by macrophages. Proc. Nat. Acad. Sci. *58*:1480-1486.

346. Imaeda, T. 1965. Electronmicroscopy. Approach to leprosy research. Int. J. Leprosy *33*:669-683.

347. Jacoby, F. 1944. A method of obtaining permanent preparations for the cytological study of pure cultures of macrophages, with special reference to their mode of division. J. Path. Bact. *56*:438-440.

348. Jacoby, F. 1965. Macrophages. *In* "Cells and Tissues in Culture," v. 2. (Ed. Willmer, E. N.) Academic Press, New York. pp. 1-93.

349. Jaffé, R. H. 1938. The reticulo-endothelial system. *In* "Handbook of Hematology," v. II. (Ed. Downey, H.) Paul B. Hoeber, Inc., New York. pp. 973-1272.

350. Jandl, J. H., Jones, A. R. and Castle, W. B. 1957. The destruction of red cells by antibodies in man. I. Observations on the sequestration and lysis of red cells altered by immune mechanisms. J. Clin. Invest. *36*:1428-1459.

351. Jandl, J. H. and Kaplan, M. E. 1960. The destruction of red cells by antibodies in man. III. Quantitative factors influencing the patterns of hemolysis *in vivo*. J. Clin. Invest. *39*:1145-1156.

352. Jandl, J. H. and Tomlinson, A. S. 1958. The destruction of red cells by antibodies in man. II. Pyrogenic, leukocytic and dermal responses to immune hemolysis. J. Clin. Invest. *37*:1202-1228.

353. Janoff, A. 1964. The role of iron in macrophages. J. Theor. Biol. *7*:168-170.

354. Jee, W. S. S. and Nolan, P. D. 1963. Origin of osteoclasts from the fusion of phagocytes. Nature *200*:225-226.

355. Jenkin, C. R. 1963. The effect of opsonins on intracellular survival of bacteria. Brit. J. Exp. Path. *44*:47-57.

356. Jenkin, C. R. and Karthigasu, K. 1962. Elimination hépatique des érythrocytes âgés et altérés chez le rat. C. R. Soc. Biol., Paris, *156*: 1006-1007.

357. Jenkin, C. R. and Rowley, D. 1963. Basis for immunity to typhoid in mice and the question of "cellular immunity." Bact. Rev. *27*:391-404.

358. Jenkin, C. R., Rowley, D. and Auzins, I. 1964. The basis for immunity to mouse typhoid. I. The carrier state. Aust. J. Exp. Biol. Med. Sci. *42*:215-228.

359. Jennings, J. F. and Hughes, L. A. 1969. Inhibition of phagocytosis by anti-macrophage antibodies. Nature *221*:79-80.

360. Jeunet, F. S., Cain, W. A. and Good, R. A. 1969. Reticuloendothelial function in the isolated perfused liver. III. Phagocytosis of *Salmonella typhosa* and *Brucella melitensis* and the blockade of the reticuloendothelial system. J. Reticuloendothel. Soc. *6*:391-410.

361. Jeunet, F. S. and Good, R. A. 1967. Reticuloendothelial function in the isolated perfused liver. I. Study of rates of clearance, role of a plasma factor, and the nature of RE blockade. J. Reticuloendothel. Soc. *4*:351-369.

362. Jeunet, F. S. and Good, R. A. 1969. Reticuloendothelial function in the isolated perfused liver. II. Phagocytosis of heat-aggregated bovine serum albumin. Demonstration of two components in the blockade of the reticuloendothelial system. J. Reticuloendothel. Soc. *6*:94-107.

363. Johnson, J. 1968. Studies on the role of the reticuloendothelial system in delayed hypersensitivity. Undergraduate honors thesis. University of Washington. Seattle, Washington.

364. Jones, A. L. 1966. The effect of polymorphonuclear leucocytes on the blastoid transformation of lymphocytes in mixed leucocyte cultures. Transplantation *4*:337-343.

365. Kajita, A., Nakamura, K., Taya, S. and Teshima, T. 1959. The electron microscopic observation on the pulmonary alveolar phagocytes of the mouse. Tohoku J. Exp. Med. *70*:311-318.

366. Kaliss, N. 1958. Immunological enhancement of tumor homografts in mice. Cancer Res. *18*:992-1003.

367. Kaliss, N. 1965. Immunological enhancement and inhibition of tumor growth: relationship to various immunological mechanisms. Fed. Proc. *24*:1024-1029.

368. Kaliss, N. 1966. Immunological enhancement: conditions for its expression and its relevance for grafts of normal tissues. Ann. N. Y. Acad. Sci. *129*:155-163.

369. Kaplan, M. H., Coons, A. H. and Deane, H. W. 1950. Localization of antigen in tissue cells. III. Cellular distribution of pneumococcal polysaccharide types II and III in the mouse. J. Exp. Med. *91*:15-29.

370. Karlsbad, G., Kessel, R. W. I., de Petris, S. and Monaco, L. 1964. Electron microscope observations of *Brucella abortus* grown within monocytes *in vitro*. J. Gen. Microbiol. *35*:383-390.

371. Karnovsky, M. L. 1961. Metabolic shifts in leucocytes during the phagocytic event. *In* "Biological Activity of the Leucocyte." (Eds. Wolstenholme, G. E. W., O'Connor, C. M., and O'Connor, M.) Ciba Fndn. Study Group No. 10; Little, Brown & Co., Boston. pp. 60-74.

372. Karnovsky, M. L. 1962. Metabolic basis of phagocytic activity. Physiol. Rev. *42*:143-168.

373. Karnovsky, M. L. and Wallach, D. F. H. 1961. The metabolic basis of phagocytosis. III. Incorporation of inorganic phosphates into various classes of phosphatides during phagocytosis. J. Biol. Chem. *236*:1895-1901.

374. Karrer, H. E. 1958. The ultrastructure of mouse lung: The alveolar macrophage. J. Biophys. and Biochem. Cytol. *4*:693-700.

375. Karrer, H. E. 1960. Electron microscopic study of the phagocytosis process in lung. J. Biophys. and Biochem. Cytol. *7*:357-366.

376. Karthigasu, K. and Jenkin, C. R. 1963. The functional development of the reticulo-endothelial system of the chick embryo. Immunology *6*:255-263.

377. Karthigasu, K., Reade, P. C. and Jenkin, C. R. 1965. The functional development of the reticulo-endothelial system. III. The bactericidal capacity of fixed macrophages of foetal and neonatal chicks and rats. Immunology *9*:67-73.

378. Kawata, H., Myrvik, Q. N. and Leake, E. S. 1964. Dissociation of tuberculin hypersensitivity as mediator for an accelerated pulmonary granulomatous response in rabbits. J. Immunol. *93*:433-438.

379. Kaye, D., Gill, F. A. and Hook, E. W. 1967. Factors influencing host resistance to *Salmonella* infections: The effects of hemolysis and erythrophagocytosis. Amer. J. Med. Sci. *254*:205-215.

380. Kessel, R. W. I. and Braun, W. 1965. Cytotoxicity of endotoxin *in vitro*. Effects on macrophages from normal guinea pigs. Aust. J. Exp. Biol. Med. Sci. *43*:511-522.

381. Kessel, R. W. I., Monaco, L. and Marchisio, M. A. 1963. The specificity of the cytotoxic action of silica—a study *in vitro*. Brit. J. Exp. Path. *44*:351-364.

382. King, E. J., Mohanty, G. P., Harrison, C. V. and Nagelschmidt, G. 1953. The action of different forms of pure silica on the lungs of rats. Brit. J. Industr. Med. *10*:9-17.

383. Konigsmark, B. W. and Sidman, R. L. 1963. Origin of brain macrophages in the mouse. J. Neuropath. Exp. Neurol. *22*:643-676.

384. Kono, Y. and Ho, M. 1965. The role of the reticuloendothelial system in interferon formation in the rabbit. Virology *25*:162-166.

385. Kossard, S. and Nelson, D. S. 1968a. Studies on cytophilic antibodies. III. Sensitization of homologous and heterologous macrophages by cytophilic antibodies: Inhibition of sensitization by normal serum. Aust. J. Exp. Biol. Med. Sci. *46*:51-61.

386. Kossard, S. and Nelson, D. S. 1968b. Studies on cytophilic antibodies. IV. The effects of proteolytic enzymes (trypsin and papain) on the attachment to macrophages of cytophilic antibodies. Aust. J. Exp. Biol. Med. Sci. *46*:63-71.

387. Kostowiecki, M. 1963. The thymic macrophages. Zeit. f. mikr. anat. Forschung *69*:585-614.

388. Kosunen, T. U., Waksman, B. H. and Samuelsson, I. K. 1963. Radioautographic study of cellular mechanisms in delayed hypersensitivity. II. Experimental allergic encephalomyelitis in the rat. J. Neuropath. Exp. Neurol. *22*:367-380.

389. Kountz, S. L., Williams, M. A., Williams, P. L., Kapros, C. and Dempster, W. J. 1963. Mechanism of rejection of homotransplanted kidneys. Nature *199*:257-260.

390. Krone, H. A. and Littig, G. 1959. Uber das Vorkammen von Schaumzellen im Stroma von Adenocarcinoma des Corpus uteri. Arch. Gynäk. *191*:432-436.

391. Landsteiner, K. and Chase, M. W. 1939. Studies on the sensitization of animals with simple chemical compounds. VI. Experiments on the sensitization of guinea pigs to poison ivy. J. Exp. Med. *69*:767-784.

392. Landsteiner, K. and Chase, M. W. 1942. Experiments on transfer of cutaneous sensitivity to simple compounds. Proc. Soc. Exp. Biol. Med. *49*:688-690.

393. Landy, M. and Braun, W. 1964. "Bacterial Endotoxins." Rutgers Intern. Symp., Quinn and Boden Co., Inc., Rahway, N. J.

394. Lang, P. G. and Ada, G. L. 1967. Antigen in tissues. IV. The effect of antibody on the retention and localization of antigen in rat lymph nodes. Immunology *13*:523-534.

395. Larsh, J. E., Jr. 1967. The present understanding on the mechanism of immunity to *Trichinella spiralis*. Amer. J. Trop. Med. Hyg. *16*:123-132.

396. Lawkowicz, W. and Krzeminska-Lawkowicz, I. 1957. "Atlas of Haematology and the Principles of Diagnosis of Blood Diseases." Polish State Med. Publ., Warsaw. 286 pp.

397. Lay, W. H. and Nussenzweig, V. 1968. Receptors for complement on leukocytes. J. Exp. Med. *128*:991-1009.

398. Leake, E. S. and Heise, E. R. 1967. Comparative cytology of alveolar and peritoneal macrophages from germ-free rats. Adv. Exp. Med. Biol. *1*:133-146.

399. Leake, E. S. and Myrvik, Q. N. 1964. Differential release of lysozyme and acid phosphatase from sub-cellular granules of normal rabbit alveolar macrophages. Brit. J. Exp. Path. *45*:384-392.

400. Leake, E. S. and Myrvik, Q. N. 1966. Digestive vacuole formation in alveolar macrophages after phagocytosis of *Mycobacterium smegmatis in vivo*. J. Reticuloendothel. Soc. *3*:83-100.

401. Leavell, B. S. and Thorup, O. A., Jr. 1960. "Fundamentals of Clinical Hematology." W. B. Saunders Co., Philadelphia. pp. 314-317.

402. Lennert, K., Caesar, R. and Müller, H. K. 1967. Electron microscopic studies of germinal centers in man. *In* "Germinal Centers in Immune Responses." (Eds. Cottier, H., Odartchenko, N., Schindler, R. and Congdon, C. C.). Springer-Verlag, New York. pp. 60-70.

403. Lewis, M. R. 1925. The formation of macrophages, epithelioid cells and giant cells from leucocytes in incubated blood. Amer. J. Path. *1*:91-100.

404. Libansky, J. 1966. The source of mononuclears at a site of inflammation. Blut *13*:20-29.

405. Liebow, A. A., Steer, A. and Billingsley, J. G. 1965. Desquamative interstitial pneumonia. Amer. J. Med. *39*:369-404.

406. LoBuglio, A. F., Cotran, R. S. and Jandl, J. H. 1967. Red cells coated with immunoglobulin G: Binding and sphering by mononuclear cells in man. Science *158*:1582-1585.

407. Loewi, G., Temple, A., Nind, A. P. P. and Axelrod, M. 1969. A study of the effects of anti-macrophage sera. Immunology *16*:99-106.

408. Low, F. N. and Freeman, J. A. 1958. "Electron Microscopic Atlas of Normal and Leukemic Human Blood." McGraw-Hill Book Co., Inc., New York. 347 pp.

409. Lumb, G. 1954. "Tumours of Lymphoid Tissue." E. and S. Livingstone Ltd., Edinburgh and London. pp. 137-141.

410. Lurie, M. B. 1960. The reticuloendothelial system, cortisone, and thyroid function: Their relation to native resistance to infection. Ann. N. Y. Acad. Sci. *88*:83-98.

411. Lurie, M. B. 1964. "Resistance to Tuberculosis: Experimental Studies in Native and Acquired Defensive Mechanisms." Harvard Univ. Press, Cambridge. 391 pp.

412. Lurie, M. B. and Dannenberg, A. M., Jr. 1965. Macrophage function in infectious disease with inbred rabbits. Bact. Rev. *29*:466-476.

413. Mackaness, G. B. 1962. Cellular resistance to infection. J. Exp. Med. *116*:381-406.

414. Mackaness, G. B. 1968. The immunology of antituberculous immunity. Amer. Rev. Resp. Dis. *97*:337-344.
415. Mackaness, G. B. and Blanden, R. V. 1967. Cellular immunity. Progr. Allergy *11*:89-140.
416. Mackaness, G. B., Blanden, R. V. and Collins, F. M. 1966. Host-parasite relations in mouse typhoid. J. Exp. Med. *124*:573-583.
417. MacKay, I. R. and Burnet, F. M. 1963. "Autoimmune Diseases. Pathogenesis, Chemistry and Therapy." Charles C Thomas, Springfield, Ill. 323 pp.
418. Maier, H. C. 1967. Lipoid pneumonia. *In* "Textbook of Medicine," 12th edition. (Eds. Beeson, P. B. and McDermott, W.) W. B. Saunders Co., Philadelphia. pp. 515-516.
419. deMan, J. C. H. 1968. Rod-like tubular structures in the cytoplasm of histiocytes in "histiocytosis X." J. Path. Bact. *95*:123-126.
420. deMan, J. C. H., Daems, W. T., Willighagen, R. G. J. and van Rijssel, T. G. 1960. Electron-dense bodies in liver tissue of the mouse in relation to the activity of acid phosphatase. J. Ultrastruct. Res. *4*:43-57.
421. Markert, C. L. 1963. Epigenetic control of specific protein synthesis in differentiating cells. *In* "Cytodifferentiation and Macromolecular Synthesis." (Ed. Locke, M.) Academic Press, New York. pp. 65-84.
422. Marshall, A. H. E. 1956. "An Outline of the Cytology and Pathology of the Reticular Tissue." Oliver and Boyd, London. pp. 23-33.
423. Matter, A., Orci, L., Forssmann, W. G. and Rouiller, Ch. 1968. The stereological analysis of the fine structure of the "micropinocytosis vermiformis" in Kupffer cells of the rat. J. Ultrastruct. Res. *23*:272-279.
424. Maximow, A. 1903. Weiteres über Entstehung, Structur und Veränderungen des Narbengewebes. Beitr. Path. Anat. u. Allgem. Path. *34*:153-188.
425. Maximow, A. A. 1924. Relation of blood cells to connective tissue and endothelium. Physiol. Rev. *4*:533-563.
426. Maximow, A. A. 1932. The macrophages or histiocytes. *In* "Special Cytology," v. 2. (Ed. Cowdry, E. V.) Paul B. Hoeber, Inc., New York. pp. 710-770.
427. Mayberry, H. E. 1964. Macrophages in post-secretory mammary involution in mice. Anat. Rec. *149*:99-111.
428. McDevitt, H. O. 1968. The cellular localization of antigen. J. Reticuloendothel. Soc. *5*:256-269.
429. McIvor, K. L. 1969. Mechanisms concerned in the contact destruction of specific target cells by alloimmune macrophages *in vitro*. Ph.D. thesis, University of Washington. Seattle, Washington.
430. McMaster, P. D. 1953. Sites of antibody formation. *In* "The Nature and Significance of the Antibody Response." (Ed. Pappenheimer, A. M., Jr.) Columbia Univ. Press, New York. pp. 13-45.
431. McMaster, P. D. and Kruse, H. 1951. The persistence in mice of cer-

tain foreign proteins and azo protein tracer-antigens derived from them. J. Exp. Med. 94:323-346.

432. Mesnil, M. A. 1895. Sur le mode de résistance des vertébrés inférieurs aux invasions microbiennes artificielles. Contribution a l'étude de l'immunite. Ann. Inst. Pasteur 9:301-351.

433. Metcalf, D., Bradley, T. R. and Robinson, W. 1967. Analysis of colonies developing in vitro from mouse bone marrow cells stimulated by kidney feeder layers or leukemic serum. J. Cell. Physiol. 69:93-108.

434. Metchnikoff, E. 1884a. Ueber eine Sprosspilzkrankheit der Daphnien. Beitrag zur Lehre über den Kampf der Phagocyten gegen Krankheitserreger. Virchow's Archiv. 96:177-195.

435. Metchnikoff, E. 1884b. Ueber die Beziehung der Phagocyten zu Milzbrandbacillen. Virchow's Archiv. 97:502-526.

436. Metchnikoff, E. 1888. Ueber die phagocytäre Rolle der Tuberkelriesenzellen. Arch. Path. Anat. Physiol. (Virchow's) 113:63-94.

437. Metchnikoff, E. 1905. "Immunity in Infective Diseases." Cambridge University Press, Boston. 591 pp.

438. Metzger, G. V. and Casarett, L. J. 1967. Some effects of divalent cations on in vitro phagocytosis. Adv. Exp. Med. Biol. 1:163-174.

439. Miescher, P. A. and Müller-Eberhard, H. J. 1968. "Textbook of Immunopathology," Vol. 1. Grune & Stratton, Inc., New York. pp. 132-188.

440. Miki, K. and Mackaness, G. B. 1964. The passive transfer of acquired resistance to Listeria monocytogenes. J. Exp. Med. 120:93-103.

440a. Mills, D. M. and Zucker-Franklin, D. 1969. Electron microscopic study of isolated Kupffer cells. Amer. J. Path. 54:147-166.

441. Mims, C. A. 1964a. Aspects of the pathogenesis of virus diseases. Bact. Rev. 28:30-71.

442. Mims, C. A. 1964b. The peritoneal macrophages of mice. Brit. J. Exp. Path. 45:37-43.

443. Mishell, R. I. and Dutton, R. W. 1966. Immunization of normal mouse spleen cell suspensions in vitro. Science 153:1004-1005.

444. Mitchison, N. A. 1955. Studies on the immunological response to foreign tumor transplants in the mouse. I. The role of lymph node cells in conferring immunity by adoptive transfer. J. Exp. Med. 102:157-177.

445. Mitchison, N. A. 1969. The immunogenic capacity of antigen taken up by peritoneal exudate cells. Immunology 16:1-14.

446. Moore, C. V. 1967. Gaucher's disease. In "Textbook of Medicine," 12th edition. (Eds. Beeson, P. B. and McDermott, W.) W. B. Saunders Co., Philadelphia. pp. 1099-1101.

447. Mizunoe, K. and Dannenberg, A. M., Jr. 1965. Hydrolases of rabbit macrophages. III. Effect of BCG vaccination, tissue culture, and ingested tubercle bacilli. Proc. Soc. Exp. Biol. Med. 120:284-290.

448. Mollo, F. and Governa, M. 1961. Richerche sperimentali sulle modificazioni iperplastiche dei linfonodi in seguito alla azione di prodotti della lisi in vitro dei macrofagi. Med. Lavoro 52:721-743.

449. Monis, B., Weinberg, T. and Spector, G. J. 1968. The carrageenan granuloma in the rat. A model for the study of the structure and function of macrophages. Brit. J. Exp. Path. 49:302-310.

450. Moore, R. D. and Schoenberg, M. D. 1964. The response of the histio-cytes and macrophages in the lungs of rabbits injected with Freund's adjuvant. Brit. J. Exp. Path. 45:488-497.

451. Moore, R. D. and Schoenberg, M. D. 1968. Restimulation of antibody synthesis by antigen in cultures of lymphocytes. Nature 219:297-298.

452. Mosier, D. E. 1967. A requirement for two cell types for antibody formation in vitro. Science 158:1573-1575.

453. Mosier, D. E. 1969. Cell interactions in the primary immune response in vitro: A requirement for specific cell clusters. J. Exp. Med. 129:351-362.

454. Muir, A. R. and Golberg, L. 1961. Observations on subcutaneous macro-phages. Phagocytosis of iron-dextran and ferritin synthesis. Quart. J. Exp. Physiol. 46:289-298.

455. Müller-Eberhard, H. J. 1968. Chemistry and reaction mechanisms of complement. Adv. Immunol. 8:1-80.

456. Murphy, J. B. 1926. The lymphocyte in resistance to tissue grafting, malignant disease, and tuberculous infection. Monogr. Rockefeller Inst. Med. Res. No. 21. pp. 123-127.

457. Myrvik, Q. N. and Evans, D. G. 1967a. Metabolic and immunologic activities of alveolar macrophages. Arch. Environ. Health 14:92-96.

458. Myrvik, Q. N. and Evans, D. G. 1967b. Effect of Bacillus-Calmette-Guerin on the metabolism of alveolar macrophages. Adv. Exp. Med. Biol. 1:203-213.

459. Myrvik, Q. N., Leake, E. S. and Fariss, B. 1961a. Pulmonary alveolar macrophages from the normal rabbit: A technique to procure them in a high state of purity. J. Immunol. 86:128-132.

460. Myrvik, Q. N., Leake, E. S. and Fariss, B. 1961b. Lysozyme content of alveolar and peritoneal macrophages from the rabbit. J. Immunol. 86:133-136.

461. Myrvik, Q. N., Leake, E. S. and Oshima, S. 1962. A study of macro-phages and epithelioid-like cells from granulomatous (BCG-in-duced) lungs of rabbits. J. Immunol. 89:745-751.

462. Nagaishi, C., Okada, Y., Ishiko, S. and Daido, S. 1964. Electron microscopic observations of the pulmonary alveoli. Exp. Med. Surg. 22:81-117.

463. Nelson, D. S. 1965. The effects of anticoagulants and other drugs on cellular and cutaneous reactions to antigen in guinea-pigs with delayed-type hypersensitivity. Immunology 9:219-234.

463a. Nelson, D. S. 1969. "Macrophages and Immunity." Frontiers of Biol-ogy, v. II. John Wiley & Sons, Inc., New York.

464. Nelson, D. S. and Boyden, S. V. 1963. The loss of macrophages from peritoneal exudates following the injection of antigen into guinea-pigs with delayed hypersensitivity. Immunology 6:264-275.

465. Nelson, D. S. and Boyden, S. V. 1967. Macrophage cytophilic antibodies and delayed hypersensitivity. Brit. Med. Bull. *23*:15-20.

466. Nelson, D. S., Kossard, S. and Cox, P. E. 1967. Heterogeneity of cytophilic antibodies in immunized mice. Experientia *23*:490-491.

467. Nelson, D. S. and Mildenhall, P. 1968. Studies on cytophilic antibodies. II. The production by guinea pigs of macrophage cytophilic antibodies to sheep erythrocytes and human serum albumin: Relationship to the production of other antibodies and the development of delayed-type hypersensitivity. Aust. J. Exp. Biol. Med. Sci. *46*: 33-49.

468. Nelson, D. S. and North, R. J. 1965. The fate of peritoneal macrophages after the injection of antigen into guinea pigs with delayed-type hypersensitivity. Lab. Invest. *14*:89-101.

469. Nelstrop, A. E., Taylor, G. and Collard, P. 1968a. Studies on phagocytosis. I. Antigen clearance studies in rabbits. Immunology *14*:325-337.

470. Nelstrop, A. E., Taylor, G. and Collard, P. 1968b. Studies on phagocytosis. II. *In vitro* phagocytosis by macrophages. Immunology *14*:339-346.

471. Nelstrop, A. E., Taylor, G. and Collard, P. 1968c. Studies on phagocytosis. III. Antigen clearance studies in invertebrates and poikilothermic vertebrates. Immunology *14*:347-356.

472. Nicol, T. and Bilbey, D. L. J. 1958. Substances depressing the phagocytic activity of the reticulo-endothelial system. Nature *182*:606.

473. Nicol, T., Bilbey, D. L. J. and Ware, C. C. 1958. Effect of various stilbene compounds on the phagocytic activity of the reticulo-endothelial system. Nature *181*:1538-1539.

474. Nicol, T. and Cordingly, J. L. 1966. Elimination via the bronchial tree of carbon stored by rat liver macrophages suggesting Kupffer cell migration. (Abstr.) J. Anat. *100*:922-923.

475. Nicol, T. and Cordingly, J. L. 1967. Reticuloendothelial excretion via the bronchial tree. Adv. Exp. Med. Biol. *1*:58-62.

476. Nicol, T., Vernon-Roberts, B. and Quantock, D. C. 1966. The effects of oestrogen: anti-oestrogen interaction on the reticulo-endothelial system and reproductive tract in ovariectomized mice. (Abstr.) J. Anat. *100*:921.

477. Niebauer, G. 1968. The melanophage (macrophage). Exp. Biol. Med. *2*:93-97.

478. Njoku-Obi, A. N. and Osebold, J. W. 1962. Studies on mechanisms of immunity in listeriosis. I. Interaction of peritoneal exudate cells from sheep with *Listeria monocytogenes in vitro*. J. Immunol. *89*:187-194.

479. Normann, S. J. and Benditt, E. P. 1965a. Function of the reticuloendothelial system. I. A study on the phenomenon of carbon clearance inhibition. J. Exp. Med. *122*:693-707.

480. Normann, S. J. and Benditt, E. P. 1965b. Function of the reticulo-

endothelial system. II. Participation of a serum factor in carbon clearance. J. Exp. Med. *122*:709-719.

481. North, R. J. 1966a. The localization by electron microscopy of nucleoside phosphatase activity in guinea pig phagocytic cells. J. Ultrastruct. Res. *16*:83-95.

482. North, R. J. 1966b. The localization by electron microscopy of acid phosphatase activity in guinea pig macrophages. J. Ultrastruct. Res. *16*:96-108.

483. North, R. J. 1968. The uptake of particulate antigens. J. Reticuloendothel. Soc. *5*:203-229.

484. North, R. J. and Mackaness, G. B. 1963a. Electronmicroscopical observations on the peritoneal macrophages of normal mice and mice immunized with *Listeria monocytogenes*. I. Structure of normal macrophages and the early cytoplasmic response to the presence of ingested bacteria. Brit. J. Exp. Path. *44*:601-607.

485. North, R. J. and Mackaness, G. B. 1963b. Electronmicroscopical observations on the peritoneal macrophages of normal mice and mice immunized with *Listeria monocytogenes*. II. Structure of macrophages from immune mice and early cytoplasmic response to the presence of ingested bacteria. Brit. J. Exp. Path. *44*:608-611.

486. Northover, B. J. 1961. The effect of histamine and 5-hydroxytryptamine on phagocytosis of staphylococci *in vitro* by polymorphs and macrophages. J. Path. Bact. *82*:355-361.

487. Norton, W. L. and Ziff, M. 1966. Electron microscopic observations on the rheumatoid synovial membrane. Arthritis Rheum. *9*:589-610.

488. Nossal, G. J. V., Abbot, A. and Mitchell, J. 1968. Antigens in immunity. XIV. Electron microscopic radioautographic studies of antigen capture in the lymph node medulla. J. Exp. Med. *127*: 263-276.

489. Nossal, G. J. V., Abbot, A., Mitchell, J. and Lummus, Z. 1968. Antigens in immunity. XV. Ultrastructural features of antigen capture in primary and secondary lymphoid follicles. J. Exp. Med. *127*: 277-289.

490. Nossal, G. J. V., Ada, G. L. and Austin, C. M. 1964a. Antigens in immunity. II. Immunogenic properties of flagella, polymerized flagellin, and flagellin in the primary response. Aust. J. Exp. Biol. Med. Sci. *42*:283-294.

491. Nossal, G. J. V., Ada, G. L. and Austin, C. M. 1964b. Antigens in immunity. IV. Cellular localization of [125]I- and ^{131}I-labelled flagella in lymph nodes. Aust. J. Exp. Biol. Med. Sci. *42*:311-330.

492. O'Grady, L. F., Lewis, J. P. and Trobaugh, F. E., Jr. 1968. The effect of erythropoietin on differentiated erythroid precursors. J. Lab. Clin. Med. *71*:693-703.

493. Old, L. J., Boyse, E. A., Bennett, B. and Lilly, F. 1963. Peritoneal cells as an immune population in transplantation studies. *In* "Cell-bound Antibodies." (Eds. Amos, D. B. and Koprowski, H.) Wistar Inst. Press, Philadelphia. pp. 89-98.

494. Old, L. J., Clarke, D. A., Benacerraf, B. and Goldsmith, M. 1960. The reticuloendothelial system and the neoplastic process. Ann. N. Y. Acad. Sci. *88*:264-280.

495. Oppenheim, J. J. 1968. Relationship of *in vitro* lymphocyte transformation to delayed hypersensitivity in guinea pigs and man. Fed. Proc. *27*:21-28.

496. Oren, R., Farnham, A. E., Saito, K., Milofsky, E. and Karnovsky, M. L. 1963. Metabolic patterns in three types of phagocytizing cells. J. Cell Biol. *17*:487-501.

497. Oshima, S., Myrvik, Q. N. and Leake, E. 1961. The demonstration of lysozyme as a dominant tuberculostatic factor in extracts of granulomatous lungs. Brit. J. Exp. Path. *42*:138-144.

498. Ouchi, E., Selvaraj, R. J. and Sbarra, A. J. 1965. The biochemical activities of rabbit alveolar macrophages during phagocytosis. Exp. Cell Res. *40*:456-468.

499. Palade, G. E. 1955. Relations between endoplasmic reticulum and the plasma membrane in macrophages. (Abstr.) Anat. Rec. *121*:445.

500. Palade, G. E. 1956. The endoplasmic reticulum. J. Biophys. Biochem. Cytol. *2*(Suppl.):85-97.

501. Panijel, J. and Cayeux, P. 1968. Immunosuppressive effects of macrophage antiserum. Immunology *14*:769-780.

502. Paradisi, E. R., de Bonaparte, Y. P. and Morgenfeld, M. C. 1968. Blasts in lepromatous leprosy. Lancet *i*:308-309.

503. Paradisi, E. R., de Bonaparte, Y. P. and Morgenfeld, M. C. 1969. Response of anergic patients to transfer of leukocytes. New Eng. J. Med. *280*:859-861.

504. Parish, W. E. 1965. Differentiation between cytophilic antibody and an opsonin by a macrophage phagocytic system. Nature *208*: 594-595.

505. Paterson, P. Y. 1968. Experimental autoimmune (allergic) encephalomyelitis. *In* "Textbook of Immunopathology," v. 1. (Eds. Miescher, P. A. and Müller-Eberhard, H. J.) Grune & Stratton, Inc., New York. pp. 132-149.

506. Pearsall, N. N. and Weiser, R. S. 1968a. The macrophage in allograft immunity. I. Effects of silica as a specific macrophage toxin. J. Reticuloendothel. Soc. *5*:107-120.

507. Pearsall, N. N. and Weiser, R. S. 1968b. The macrophage in allograft immunity. II. Passive transfer with immune macrophages. J. Reticuloendothel. Soc. *5*:121-133.

508. Perkins, E. H. and Leonard, M. R. 1963. Specificity of phagocytosis as it may relate to antibody formation. J. Immunol. *90*:228, 237.

509. Perkins, E. H., Nettesheim, P., Morita, T. and Walburg, H. E., Jr. 1967. The engulfing potential of peritoneal phagocytes of conventional and germ-free mice. Adv. Exp. Med. Biol. *1*:175-187.

510. Pernis, B. 1955. Studi chimico-biologici sullo ialino della silicosi. I: Sul contenuto in proteine fibrose (collageno ed elastina). Med. Lavoro *46*:659-667.

511. Pernis, B., Bairati, A. and Milanesi, S. 1966. Cellular and humoral reactions to Freund's adjuvant in guinea pigs. Path. Microbiol. 29:837-853.

512. Persellin, R. H. and Ziff, M. 1966. The effect of gold salt on lysosomal enzymes of the peritoneal macrophage. Arthritis Rheum. 9:57-65.

513. Pettersen, J. C. 1964. A comparison of the metalophilic reticuloendothelial cells to cells containing acid phosphatase and non-specific esterase in the lymphoid nodules of normal and stimulated rat spleens. Anat. Rec. 149:269-277.

514. Phadke, A. M. and Phadke, G. M. 1961. Occurrence of macrophage cells in the semen and in the epididymis in cases of male infertility. J. Reprod. Fertil. 2:400-403.

515. Pinchuck, P., Fishman, M., Adler, F. L. and Maurer, P. H. 1968. Antibody formation: Initiation in "nonresponder" mice by macrophage synthetic polypeptide RNA. Science 160:194-195.

516. Pinkett, M. O., Cowdrey, C. R. and Nowell, P. C. 1966. Mixed hematopoietic and pulmonary origin of "alveolar macrophages" as demonstrated by chromosome markers. Amer. J. Path. 48:859-867.

517. Pisano, J. C., Filkins, J. P. and DiLuzio, N. R. 1967. Development and evaluation of a method for the isolation of Kupffer cells. (Abstr.) J. Reticuloendothel. Soc. 4:431-432.

518. Pisano, J. C., Patterson, J. T. and DiLuzio, N. R. 1968. Reticuloendothelial blockade: Effect of puromycin on opsonin-dependent recovery. Science 162:565-567.

519. Pluznik, D. H. and Sachs, L. 1966. The induction of clones of normal "mast" cells by a substance from conditioned medium. Exp. Cell Res. 43:553-563.

520. Pogo, B. G. T., Allfrey, V. G. and Mirsky, A. E. 1966. RNA synthesis and histone acetylation during the course of gene activation in lymphocytes. Proc. Nat. Acad. Sci. 55:805-812.

521. Policard, A. 1957. The morphology and physiology of the reticulohistiocytic cell. In "Physiopathology of the Reticulo-endothelial System." (Eds. Halpern, B. N., Benacerraf, B. and Delafresnaye, J. F.) Blackwell Scientific Publications, Oxford. pp. 12-25.

522. Policard, A. and Bessis, M. 1953. Fractionnement d'hématies par les leucocytes au cours de leur phagocytose. C. R. Soc. Biol. (Paris) 147:982-984.

523. Policard, A. and Bessis, M. 1958. Sur un mode d'incorporation des macromolécules par la cellule, visible au microscope électronique: la rhophéocytose. C. R. Acad. Sci. (Paris) 246:3194-3197.

524. Policard, A., Collet, A. and Pregermain, S. 1957. Electron microscopic studies on alveolar cells from mammals. In "Electron Microscopy." (Eds. Sjostrand, F. S. and Rhodin, J.) Academic Press, New York. pp. 244-246.

525. Pomales-Lebron, A. and Stinebring, W. R. 1957. Intracellular multiplication of Brucella abortus in normal and immune mononuclear phagocytes. Proc. Soc. Exp. Biol. Med. 94:78-83.

526. Prehn, R. T. and Main, J. M. 1957. Immunity to methylcholanthrene-induced sarcomas. J. Nat. Cancer Inst. *18*:769-778.

527. Pribnow, J. F. and Silverman, M. S. 1967. Studies on the radio-sensitive phase of the primary antibody response in rabbits. I. The role of the macrophage. J. Immunol. *98*:225-229.

528. Propp, R. P. and Alper, C. A. 1968. C'3 synthesis in human fetus and lack of transplacental passage. Science *162*:672-673.

529. Rabiner, S. F. and Friedman, L. H. 1968. The role of intravascular haemolysis and the reticulo-endothelial system in the production of a hypercoagulable state. Brit. J. Haemat. *14*:105-118.

530. Rabinovich, M. 1967. The dissociation of the attachment and ingestion phases of phagocytosis by macrophages. Exp. Cell Res. *46*:19-28.

531. Rabinovitch, M. 1968. Effect of antiserum on the attachment of modified erythrocytes to normal or to trypsinized macrophages. Proc. Soc. Exp. Biol. Med. *127*:351-355.

532. Rabinovitch, M. and Gary, P. P. 1968. Effect of the uptake of staphylococci on the ingestion of glutaraldehyde-treated red cells attached to macrophages. Exp. Cell Res. *52*:363-369.

533. Rabinowitz, Y. and Schrek, R. 1962. "Monocytic" cells of normal blood, Schilling and Naegeli leukemia, and leukemic reticuloendotheliosis in slide chambers. Blood *20*:453-470.

534. Raffel, S. 1961. "Immunity," 2nd edition. Appleton-Century-Crofts, Inc., New York. pp. 430-432.

535. Ralston, D. J. and Elberg, S. S. 1969. Serum-mediated immune cellular responses to *Brucella melitensis* REV I. II. Restriction of *Brucella* by immune sera and macrophages. J. Reticuloendothel. Soc. *6*:109-139.

536. Ransom, J. P., Pasternak, V. Z. and Heller, J. H. 1962. Effect of a reticuloendothelial stimulating agent (Restim) on resistance of mice. J. Bact. *84*:466-472.

537. Ravin, H. A., Rowley, D., Jenkins, C. and Fine, J. 1960. On the absorption of bacterial endotoxin from the gastro-intestinal tract of the normal and shocked animal. J. Exp. Med. *112*:783-792.

538. Reade, P. C. 1968. The development of bactericidal activity in rat peritoneal macrophages. Aust. J. Exp. Biol. Med. Sci. *46*:231-247.

539. Reade, P. C. and Casley-Smith, J. R. 1965. The functional development of the reticulo-endothelial system. II. The histology of blood clearance by the fixed macrophages of foetal rats. Immunology *9*:61-66.

540. Reade, P. C. and Jenkin, C. R. 1965. The functional development of the reticulo-endothelial system. I. The uptake of intravenously injected particles by foetal rats. Immunology *9*:53-60.

541. Rebuck, J. W. and Crowley, J. H. 1955. A method of studying leukocytic functions *in vivo*. Ann. N. Y. Acad. Sci. *59*:757-805.

542. Rebuck, J. W. and Lo Grippo, G. A. 1961. Characteristics and interrelationships of the various cells in the RE cell, macrophage, lymphocyte and plasma cell series in man. Lab. Invest. *10*:1068-1093.

543. Rebuck, J. W., Whitehouse, F. W. and Noonan, S. M. 1967. A major fault in diabetic inflammation: Failure of leukocytic glycogen transfer to histiocytes. Adv. Exp. Med. Biol. *1*:369-381.

544. Rees, R. J. W. 1964. The significance of the lepromin reaction in man. Progr. Allergy *8*:224-258.

545. Rees, R. J. W., Waters, M. F. R., Weddell, A. G. M. and Palmer, E. 1967. Experimental lepromatous leprosy. Nature *215*:599-602.

546. Reid, J. D. and Mackay, J. B. 1967a. The role of delayed hypersensitivity in granulomatous reactions to mycobacteria: 1. Relationship of delayed reaction size to severity of granulomatous reactions after intradermal injections of mycobacteria. Tubercle *48*:100-108.

547. Reid, J. D. and Mackay, J. B. 1967b. The role of delayed hypersensitivity in granulomatous reactions to mycobacteria: 2. Reactions to intradermal injections of intact and disintegrated organisms. Tubercle *48*:109-113.

548. Rich, A. R. 1951a. "The Pathogenesis of Tuberculosis." Charles C Thomas, Springfield, Ill. pp. 716-726.

549. Rich, A. R. 1951b. "The Pathogenesis of Tuberculosis." Charles C Thomas, Springfield, Ill. pp. 515-562.

550. Richter, K. M. 1958. Some *in vitro* and *in vivo* studies on several mesenchymal cell types bearing on the problem of the reticuloendothelial system. Ann. N. Y. Acad. Sci. *73*:139-185.

551. Ridley, D. S. and Jopling, W. H. 1966. Classification of leprosy according to immunity. Int. J. Leprosy *34*:255-273.

552. Robertson, O. H. 1941. Phagocytosis of foreign material in the lung. Physiol. Rev. *21*:112-139.

553. Rose, N. R. 1965. Autoimmune diseases. *In* "The Inflammatory Process." (Eds. Zweifach, B. W., Grant, L. and McCluskey, R. T.) Academic Press, New York. pp. 731-762.

554. Roser, B. 1965. The distribution of intravenously injected peritoneal macrophages in the mouse. Aust. J. Exp. Biol. Med. Sci. *43*:553-562.

555. Roser, B. 1968. The distribution of intravenously injected Kupffer cells in the mouse. J. Reticuloendothel. Soc. *5*:455-471.

556. Ross, R. 1964. Studies of collagen formation in healing wounds. Adv. Biol. Skin *5*:144-164.

557. Rouiller, C. 1962. *In* "Aktuelle Probleme der Hepatologie." (Eds. Martini, G. A. and Sherlock, S.) Second Symp. Int. Assoc. for the Study of the Liver. Georg Thieme Verlag, Stuttgart. pp. 1-8.

558. Rous, P. 1923. Destruction of the red blood corpuscles in health and disease. Physiol. Rev. *3*:75-105.

559. Rous, P. and Beard, J. W. 1934. Selection with the magnet and cultivation of reticulo-endothelial cells (Kupffer cells). J. Exp. Med. *59*:577-591.

560. Rowley, D. 1962. Phagocytosis. Adv. Immunol. *2*:241-264.

561. Rowley, D. and Leuchtenberger, C. 1964. Antigen-stimulated desoxyribonucleic-acid synthesis *in vitro* by sensitized mouse macrophages. Lancet *ii*:734-735.

562. Rowley, D., Turner, K. J. and Jenkin, C. R. 1964. The basis for immunity to mouse typhoid. 3. Cell-bound antibody. Aust. J. Exp. Biol. Med. Sci. *42*:237-248.

563. Rubin, E. 1964. Studies in hepatic reticuloendothelial function and proliferation with tritiated thymidine. (Abstr.) J. Reticuloendothel. Soc. *1*:345-346.

564. Russell, P. and Roser, B. 1966. The distribution and behavior of intravenously injected pulmonary alveolar macrophages in the mouse. Aust. J. Exp. Biol. Med. Sci. *44*:629-637.

565. Russell, P. S. and Monaco, A. P. 1964. "The Biology of Tissue Transplantation." Little, Brown & Co., Boston. 207 pp.

566. Rutenburg, S. H., Schweinburg, F. B. and Fine, J. 1960. *In vitro* detoxification of bacterial endotoxin by macrophages. J. Exp. Med. *112*:801-807.

567. Saba, T. M. and DiLuzio, N. R. 1968. Evaluation of humoral and cellular mechanisms of methyl palmitate induced reticuloendothelial depression. Life Sci. *7*:337-347.

568. Sabin, F. R. 1939. Cellular reactions to a dye-protein with a concept of the mechanism of antibody formation. J. Exp. Med. *70*: 67-83.

569. Sabin, F. R. and Doan, C. A. 1926. The presence of desquamated endothelial cells, the so-called clasmatocytes, in normal mammalian blood. J. Exp. Med. *43*:823-838.

570. Sacks, B. 1926. The reticulo-endothelial system. Physiol. Rev. *6*:504-545.

571. St. George, S. 1960. Separation of reticuloendothelial and parenchymal cells of rat's liver by a new gentle technique. *In* "Reticuloendothelial Structure and Function." (Ed. Heller, J. H.), Ronald Press, New York. pp. 449-461.

572. Saito, K., Nakano, M., Akiyama, T. and Ushiba, D. 1962. Passive transfer of immunity to typhoid by macrophages. J. Bact. *84*:500-507.

573. Saito, K. and Suter, E. 1965. Lysosomal acid hydrolases in mice infected with BCG. J. Exp. Med. *121*:727-738.

574. Salky, N. K., Mills, D. and DiLuzio, N. R. 1965. Activity of the reticuloendothelial system in diseases of altered immunity. J. Lab. Clin. Med. *66*:952-960.

575. Salm, R. 1962. Macrophages in endometrial lesions. J. Path. Bact. *83*:405-409.

576. Schoenberg, M. D., Mumaw, V. R., Moore, R. D. and Weisberger, A. S. 1964. Cytoplasmic interaction between macrophages and lymphocytic cells in antibody synthesis. Science *143*:964-965.

577. Schowengerdt, C. G., Suyemoto, R. and Main, F. B. 1969. Granulomatous and fibrous mediastinitis. A review and analysis of 180 cases. J. Thorac. Cardiov. Surg. *57*:365-379.

578. Schwab, J. H. and Ohanian, S. H. 1967. Degradation of streptococcal cell wall antigens *in vivo*. J. Bact. *94*:1346-1352.

579. Schweinburg, F. B. and Fine, J. 1960. Evidence for a lethal endotoxemia as the fundamental feature of irreversibility in three types
of traumatic shock. J. Exp. Med. *112*:793-800.

580. Scully, R. E. and Richardson, G. S. 1961. Luteinization of the stroma
of metastatic cancer involving the ovary and its endocrine significance. Cancer *14*:827-840.

581. Sela, M. 1966. Immunologic studies with synthetic polypeptides. Adv.
Immunol. *5*:30-129.

582. Sever, J. L. 1960. Passive transfer of resistance to tuberculosis through
use of monocytes. Proc. Soc. Exp. Biol. Med. *103*:326-329.

583. Sharp, J. A. and Burwell, R. G. 1960. Interaction ("peripolesis") of
macrophages and lymphocytes after skin homografting or challenge
with soluble antigens. Nature *188*:474-475.

584. Sheagren, J. N., Block, J. B., Trautman, J. R. and Wolff, S. M. 1969.
Immunologic reactivity in patients with leprosy. Ann. Intern. Med.
70:295-302.

585. Shepard, C. C. 1960. The experimental disease that follows the injection of human leprosy bacilli into the footpads of mice. J.
Exp. Med. *112*:445-454.

586. Sherwin, R. P., Richters, V., Brooks, M. and Buckley, R. D. 1968. The
phenomenon of macrophage congregation *in vitro* and its relationship to *in vivo* NO$_2$ exposure of guinea pigs. Lab. Invest. *18*:
269-277.

587. Shorter, R. G., Titus, J. L. and Divertie, M. B. 1964. Cell turnover
in the respiratory tract. Dis. Chest *46*:138-142.

588. Silverman, L. and Shorter, R. G. 1963. Histogenesis of the multinucleated giant cell. Lab. Invest. *12*:985-990.

589. Simar, L., Betz, E. H. and Lejeune, G. 1967. Ultrastructural modifi-
cations of the lymph nodes after homologous skin grafting in the
mouse. *In* "Germinal Centers in Immune Responses." (Eds.
Cottier, H., Odartchenko, N., Schindler, R. and Congdon, C. C.)
Springer-Verlag, New York. pp. 60-70.

590. Simpson, C. L. 1952. Trypan blue-induced tumours of rats. Brit. J.
Exp. Path. *33*:524-528.

591. Singer, J. M., Lavie, S., Adlersberg, L., Ende, E., Hoenig, E. M. and
Tchorsh, Y. 1967. The use of radioiodinated latex particles for
in vivo studies of phagocytosis. Adv. Exp. Med. Biol. *1*:18-24.

592. Smith, R. T. 1968. Tumor-specific immune mechanisms. New Eng. J.
Med. *278*:1207-1214; 1268-1275.

593. Smith, T. J. and Wagner, R. R. 1967a. Rabbit macrophage interferons.
I. Conditions for biosynthesis by virus-infected and uninfected cells.
J. Exp. Med. *125*:559-577.

594. Smith, T. J. and Wagner, R. R. 1967b. Rabbit macrophage interferons.
II. Some physicochemical properties and estimations of molecular
weights. J. Exp. Med. *125*:579-593.

595. Smithers, S. R. 1967. The induction and nature of antibody response
to parasites. *In* "Immunologic Aspects of Parasitic Infections." Pan

American Health Organization, Scientific Publication No. 150, pp. 43-49.

596. Snell, J. F. 1960. The reticuloendothelial system: I. Chemical methods of stimulation of the reticuloendothelial system. Ann. N. Y. Acad. Sci. *88*:56-77.

597. Snodgrass, M. J. 1968. A study of some histochemical and phagocytic reactions of the sinus lining cells of the rabbit's spleen. Anat. Rec. *161*:353-360.

598. Sorokin, S. P. 1966. A morphologic and cytochemical study on the great alveolar cell. J. Histochem. Cytochem. *14*:884-897.

599. Soulsby, E. J. L. 1967. Lymphocyte, macrophage and other cell reactions to parasites. *In* "Immunologic Aspects of Parasitic Infections." Pan American Health Organization, Scientific Publication No. 150, pp. 66-90.

600. Spaet, T. H., Horowitz, H. I., Zucker-Franklin, D., Cintron, J. and Biezenski, J. J. 1961. Reticuloendothelial clearance of blood thromboplastin by rats. Blood *17*:196-205.

601. Spain, D. M., Molomut, M. N. and Haber, A. 1950. Biological studies on cortisone in mice. Science *112*:335-337.

602. Spector, W. G. 1967. Histology of allergic inflammation. Brit. Med. Bull. *23*:35-38.

603. Spector, W. G. and Coote, E. 1965. Differentially labelled blood cells in the reaction to paraffin oil. J. Path. Bact. *90*:589-598.

604. Spector, W. G., Walters, M. N. and Willoughby, D. A. 1965. The origin of the mononuclear cells in inflammatory exudates induced by fibrinogen. J. Path. Bact. *90*:181-192.

605. Spector, W. G. and Willoughby, D. A. 1968. The origin of mononuclear cells in chronic inflammation and tuberculin reactions in the rat. J. Path. Bact. *96*:389-399.

606. Spencer, H. and Shorter, R. G. 1962. Cell turnover in pulmonary tissues. Nature *194*:880.

607. Stanley, N. F. 1949. Studies on *Listeria monocytogenes*. I. Isolation of a monocytosis-producing agent (MPA). Aust. J. Exp. Biol. Med. Sci. *27*:123-131.

608. Stanley, N. F. 1950. The augmenting action of lecithin and the lipoids of *Aspergillus fumigatus* and *Listeria monocytogenes* in antibody production using *Salmonella typhi-murium* as an antigen. Aust. J. Exp. Biol. Med. Sci. *28*:109-115.

609. Stecher, V. J. and Thorbecke, G. J. 1967a. Sites of synthesis of serum proteins. I. Serum proteins produced by macrophages *in vitro*. J. Immunol. *99*:643-652.

610. Stecher, V. J. and Thorbecke, G. J. 1967b. Sites of synthesis of serum proteins. II. Medium requirements for serum protein production by rat macrophages. J. Immunol. *99*:653-659.

611. Stevens, K. M. and McKenna, J. M. 1958. Studies on antibody synthesis initiated *in vitro*. J. Exp. Med. *107*:537-559.

612. Stinebring, W. R. and Youngner, J. S. 1964. Patterns of interferon appearance in mice injected with bacteria or bacterial endotoxin. Nature 204:712.

613. Storb, U. and Weiser, R. S. 1968. Kinetics of mouse spleen cell populations during the immune response. J. Reticuloendothel. Soc. 5:81-106.

614. Stuart, A. E. 1963. Structural and functional effects of lipids on the reticulo-endothelial system. Colloques internationaux du C.N.R.S. 115:129-142.

615. Stuart, A. E. 1967. The role of the environment in determining the discriminatory activity of the human phagocytic cell. Adv. Exp. Med. Biol. 1:147-162.

616. Stuart, A. E. 1968. The reticulo-endothelial apparatus of the lesser octopus, Eledone cirrosa. J. Path. Bact. 96:401-412.

617. Stuart, A. E. and Davidson, A. E. 1964. Effect of simple lipids on antibody formation after injection of foreign red cells. J. Path. Bact. 87:305-316.

618. Sulitzeanu, D. 1968. Affinity of antigen for white cells and its relation to the induction of antibody formation. Bact. Rev. 32:404-424.

619. Suter, E. and Ramseier, H. 1964. Cellular reactions in infection. Adv. Immunol. 4:117-173.

620. Sutton, J. S. and Weiss, L. 1966. Transformation of monocytes in tissue culture into macrophages, epithelioid cells, and multinucleated giant cells. An electron microscope study. J. Cell Biol. 28:303-332.

621. Svejcar, J. and Johanovsky, J. 1961a. Demonstration of delayed (tuberculin) type hypersensitivity in vitro. I. Selection of methods. Z. Immunitat. 122:398-419.

622. Svejcar, J. and Johanovsky, J. 1961b. Demonstration of delayed (tuberculin) type hypersensitivity in vitro. II. Specific reaction of hypersensitive cells with antigen. Z. Immunitat. 122:420-436.

623. Svejcar, J. and Johanovsky, J. 1961c. Demonstration of delayed (tuberculin) type hypersensitivity in vitro. III. Growth stimulation of sensitive peritoneal exudate cells in antigen-containing medium. Z. Immunitat. 122:437-452.

624. Swartzendruber, D. C. 1964. Phagocytized plasma cells in mouse spleen observed by light and electron microscopy. Blood 24:432-442.

625. Swartzendruber, D. C. 1967. Observations on the ultrastructure of lymphatic tissue germinal centers. In "Germinal Centers in Immune Responses." (Eds. Cottier, H., Odartchenko, N., Schindler, R. and Congdon, C. C.) Springer-Verlag, New York. pp. 71-76.

626. Swartzendruber, D. C. and Congdon, C. C. 1963. Electron microscope observations on tingible body macrophages in mouse spleen. J. Cell Biol. 19:641-646.

627. Szakal, A. K. and Hanna, M. G., Jr. 1968. The ultrastructure of antigen localization and virus-like particles in mouse spleen germinal centers. Exp. Molec. Path. 8:75-89.

628. Tao, T. and Uhr, J. W. 1966. Primary-type antibody response *in vitro*. Science *151*:1096-1098.

629. Thompson, R. B. 1961. "Haematology." J. B. Lippincott Co., Philadelphia. pp. 99-113.

630. Thor, D. E. 1968. Human delayed hypersensitivity: an *in vitro* correlate and transfer by an RNA extract. Fed. Proc. *27*:16-20.

631. Thor, D. E. and Dray, S. 1968a. A correlate of human delayed hypersensitivity: Specific inhibition of capillary tube migration of sensitized human lymph node cells by tuberculin and histoplasmin. J. Immunol. *101*:51-61.

632. Thor, D. E. and Dray, S. 1968b. The cell-migration-inhibition correlate of delayed hypersensitivity. Conversion of human nonsensitive lymph node cells to sensitive cells with an RNA extract. J. Immunol. *101*:469-480.

633. Thorbecke, G. J. and Benacerraf, B. 1962. The reticulo-endothelial system and immunological phenomena. Progr. Allergy *6*:559-598.

634. Tompkins, E. H. 1946. Reaction of the reticuloendothelial cells to subcutaneous injections of cholesterol. Arch. Path. *42*:299-319.

635. Tompkins, E. H. 1955. The monocyte. Ann. N. Y. Acad. Sci. *59*: 732-745.

636. Tonna, E. A. 1963. Origin of osteoclasts from the fusion of phagocytes. Nature *200*:226-227.

637. Trentin, J., Wolf, N., Cheng, V., Fahlberg, W., Weiss, D. and Bonhag, R. 1967. Antibody production by mice repopulated with limited numbers of clones of lymphoid cell precursors. J. Immunol. *98*: 1326-1337.

638. Trepel, F. and Begemann, H. 1966. On the origin of the skin window macrophages. Acta Haemat. *36*:386-398.

639. Trowell, O. A. 1965. Lymphocytes. *In* "Cells and Tissues in Culture." (Ed. Willmer, E. N.) Academic Press, New York. pp. 96-172.

640. Truex, R. C. 1959. "Human Neuroanatomy." Williams & Wilkins Co., Baltimore. pp. 128-129.

641. Tsoi, M. S. and Weiser, R. S. 1968a. Mechanisms of immunity to Sarcoma I allografts in the C57BL/Ks mouse. I. Passive transfer studies with immune peritoneal macrophages in X-irradiated hosts. J. Nat. Cancer Inst. *40*:23-30.

642. Tsoi, M. S. and Weiser, R. S. 1968b. Mechanisms of immunity to Sarcoma I allografts in the C57BL/Ks mouse. II. Passive transfer studies with immune serum in X-irradiated hosts. J. Nat. Cancer Inst. *40*:31-36.

643. Tsoi, M. S. and Weiser, R. S. 1968c. Mechanisms of immunity to Sarcoma I allografts in the C57BL/Ks mouse. III. The additive and synergistic actions of macrophages and immune serum. J. Nat. Cancer Inst. *40*:37-42.

644. Tucker, D. N., Hill, W. C. and Gifford, G. E. 1963. The effect of

pH on phagocytosis by rabbit mononuclear phagocytes. J. Infect. Dis. *112*:47-52.

645. Tullis, J. L. and Surgenor, D. M. 1956. Phagocytosis-promoting factor of plasma and serum. Ann. N. Y. Acad. Sci. *66*:386-390.

646. Turk, J. L. 1967. "Delayed Hypersensitivity." Frontiers of Biology, v. 4. John Wiley & Sons, Inc., New York.

647. Turk, J. L., Heather, C. J. and Diengdoh, J. V. 1966. A histochemical analysis of mononuclear cell infiltrates of the skin with particular reference to delayed hypersensitivity in the guinea pig. Int. Arch. Allergy *29*:278-289.

648. Turk, J. L. and Polák, L. 1967. Studies on the origin and reactive ability *in vivo* of peritoneal exudate cells in delayed hypersensitivity. Int. Arch. Allergy *31*:403-416.

649. Turner, K. J., Jenkin, C. R. and Rowley, D. 1964. The basis for immunity to mouse typhoid. 2. Antibody formation during the carrier state. Aust. J. Exp. Biol. Med. Sci. *42*:229-236.

650. Uhr, J. W. 1965. Passive sensitization of lymphocytes and macrophages by antigen-antibody complexes. Proc. Nat. Acad. Sci. *54*:1599-1606.

651. Uhr, J. W. 1966. Delayed hypersensitivity. Physiol. Rev. *46*:359-419.

652. Unanue, E. R. 1968. Properties and some uses of anti-macrophage antibodies. Nature *218*:36-38.

653. Unanue, E. R. and Askonas, B. A. 1968. Persistence of immunogenicity of antigen after uptake by macrophages. J. Exp. Med. *127*:915-926.

654. Vatter, A. E., Reiss, O. K., Newman, J. K., Lindquist, K. and Groeneboer, E. 1968. Enzymes of the lung. I. Detection of esterase with a new cytochemical method. J. Cell Biol. *38*:80-98.

655. Vaughan, R. B. 1965. The discriminative behavior of rabbit phagocytes. Brit. J. Exp. Path. *46*:71-81.

656. Vaughan, R. B. and Boyden, S. V. 1964. Interactions of macrophages and erythrocytes. Immunology *7*:118-126.

657. Vigliani, E. C. and Pernis, B. 1961. The pathogenesis of silicosis: A review. Bull. Hyg. *36*:1-9.

658. Vigliani, E. C. and Pernis, B. 1963. Immunological aspects of silicosis. Adv. Tuberc. Res. *12*:230-279.

659. Virchow, R. 1885. Der Kampf der Zellen und der Bakterien. Virchow's Archiv. *101*:1-13.

660. Virolainen, M. and Defendi, V. 1967. Dependence of macrophage growth *in vitro* upon interaction with other cell types. *In* "Growth Regulating Substances for Animal Cells in Culture." (Eds. Defendi, V. and Stoker, M.) Wistar Press, Philadelphia. pp. 67-83.

661. Virolainen, M. and Defendi, V. 1968. Ability of haematopoietic spleen colonies to form macrophages *in vitro*. Nature *217*:1069-1070.

662. Volkman, A. 1966. The origin and turnover of mononuclear cells in peritoneal exudates in rats. J. Exp. Med. *124*:241-254.

663. Volkman, A. and Gowans, J. L. 1965a. The production of macro-phages in the rat. Brit. J. Exp. Path. 46:50-61.

664. Volkman, A. and Gowans, J. L. 1965b. The origin of macrophages from bone marrow in the rat. Brit. J. Exp. Path. 46:62-70.

665. Waksman, B. H. 1959. Experimental allergic encephalomyelitis and the "auto-allergic" diseases. Int. Arch. Allerg. (Suppl.) 14:1-87.

666. Waksman, B. H. 1960. The distribution of experimental auto-allergic lesions: Its relation to the distribution of small veins. Amer. J. Path. 37:673-693.

667. Waksman, B. H. 1963. The pattern of rejection in rat skin homografts and its relation to the vascular network. Lab. Invest. 12:46-57.

668. Waksman, B. H. and Matoltsy, M. 1958. The effect of tuberculin on peritoneal exudate cells of sensitized guinea pigs in surviving cell culture. J. Immunol. 81:220-234.

669. Waldorf, D. S., Sheagren, J. N., Trautman, J. R. and Block, J. B. 1966. Impaired delayed hypersensitivity in patients with lepromatous leprosy. Lancet ii:773-776.

670. Walter, J. B. and Israel, M. S. 1963. "General Pathology." Little, Brown & Co., Boston. pp. 551.

671. Ward, P. A. 1968. Chemotaxis of mononuclear cells. J. Exp. Med. 128:1201-1221.

672. Ward, P. A. and David, J. R. 1969. A leukotactic factor produced by sensitized lymphocytes. Fed. Proc. 28:630.

673. Wardlaw, A. C. and Howard, J. G. 1959. A comparative survey of the phagocytosis of different species of bacteria by Kupffer cells. Perfusion studies with the isolated rat liver. Brit. J. Exp. Path. 40:113-117.

674. Weaver, J. N. 1958. Destruction of mouse ascites tumor cells in vivo and in vitro by homologous macrophages, lymphocytes and cell-free antibodies. Proc. Amer. Assoc. Cancer Res. 2:354.

675. Weed, R. I. and Reed, C. F. 1966. Membrane alterations leading to red cell destruction. Amer. J. Med. 41:681-698.

676. Weiser, R. S., Granger, G. A., Brown, W., Baker, P., Jutila, J. and Holmes, B. 1965. Production of an acute allogenic disease in mice. Transplantation 3:10-21.

677. Weiser, R. S., Heise, E., McIvor, K., Han, S. H. and Granger, G. A. 1969. In vitro activities of immune macrophages. In "Cellular Recognition." (Eds. Smith, R. T. and Good, R. A.) Appleton-Century-Crofts, New York. pp. 215-219.

678. Weiser, R. S., Myrvik, Q. N. and Pearsall, N. N. 1969. "Fundamentals of Immunology for Students of Medicine and Related Sciences." Lea & Febiger, Philadelphia. 363 pp.

679. Weissman, G. 1966. Lysosomes and joint disease. Arthritis Rheum. 9:834-840.

680. Wiener, J. 1967. Fine structural aspects of reticuloendothelial block-ade. Adv. Exp. Med. Biol. 1:85-97.

681. Wiener, J., Spiro, D. and Russell, P. S. 1964. An electron microscopic study of the homograft reaction. Amer. J. Path. *44*:319-347.

682. Wilkins, D. J. 1967. Interaction of charged colloids with the RES. Adv. Exp. Med. Biol. *1*:25-33.

683. Wilkinson, P. C. and White, R. G. 1966. The role of mycobacteria and silica in the immunological response of the guinea pig. Immunology *11*:229-241.

684. Willoughby, D. A., Coote, E. and Spector, W. G. 1967. A monocytogenic humoral factor released after lymph node stimulation. Immunology *12*:165-178.

685. Windle, W. F., Chambers, W. W., Ricker, W. A., Ginger, L. G. and Koenig, H. 1950. Reaction of tissues to administration of a pyrogenic preparation from a *Pseudomonas* species. Amer. J. Med. Sci. *219*:422-426.

686. Windle, W. F., Littrell, J. L., Smart, J. O. and Agnew, W. 1954. Central nervous regeneration in animals in relation to observations in a human subject. (Abstr.) Anat. Rec. *118*:369-370.

687. Wintrobe, M. M. 1967. "Clinical Hematology," 6th edition. Lea & Febiger, Philadelphia. pp. 129-138.

688. Wiznitzer, T., Better, N., Rachlin, W., Atkins, N., Frank, E. D. and Fine, J. 1960. *In vivo* detoxification of endotoxin by the reticuloendothelial system. J. Exp. Med. *112*:1157-1166.

689. Wolf, A. 1969. The activity of cell-free tumour fractions in inducing immunity across a weak histocompatibility barrier. Transplantation *7*:49-58.

690. Wooles, W. R. and DiLuzio, N. R. 1964. Inhibition of homograft acceptance and homo- and heterograft rejection in chimeras by reticuloendothelial system stimulation. Proc. Soc. Exp. Biol. Med. *115*:756-759.

691. Wulff, H. R. 1962. Histochemical studies of leukocytes from an inflammatory exudate. Glycogen and phosphorylase. Acta Haemat. (Basel) *28*:86-94.

692. Wulff, H. R. 1963a. Histochemical studies of leukocytes from an inflammatory exudate. II. Succinic dehydrogenase, mitochondrial α-glycerophosphate dehydrogenase, and di- and triphosphopyridine nucleotide diaphorases. Acta Haemat. (Basel) *29*:208-217.

693. Wulff, H. R. 1963b. Histochemical studies of leukocytes from an inflammatory exudate. III. Di- and triphosphopyridine nucleotide-linked dehydrogenases. Acta Haemat. (Basel) *30*:16-24.

694. Wulff, H. R. 1963c. Histochemical studies of leukocytes from an inflammatory exudate. IV. Uridine diphosphate glucose-glycogen transglycolase. Acta Haemat. (Basel) *30*:123-127.

695. Wulff, H. R. 1963d. Histochemical studies of leukocytes from an inflammatory exudate. V. Alkaline and acid phosphatases and esterases. Acta Haemat. (Basel) *30*:159-167.

696. Wyllie, J. C., Haust, M. D. and More, R. H. 1966. The fine structure of synovial lining cells in rheumatoid arthritis. Lab. Invest. *15*:519-529.

697. Yam, L. T., Finkel, H. E., Weintraub, L. R. and Crosby, W. H. 1968. Circulating iron-containing macrophages in hemochromatosis. New Eng. J. Med. *279*:512-514.

698. Yoffey, J. M., Thomas, D. B., Moffatt, D. J., Sutherland, I. H. and Rosse, C. 1961. Non-immunological functions of the lymphocyte. *In* "Biological Activity of the Leucocyte." Ciba Fndn. Study Group No. 10. (Eds. Wolstenholme, G. E. W. and O'Connor, M.) Little, Brown & Co., Boston. pp. 45-54.

699. Youmans, G. P. and Youmans, A. S. 1969. Recent studies on acquired immunity in tuberculosis. Current Topics in Microbiology and Immunol. *48*:129-178.

Index

ACUTE allogeneic disease (AAD), 118
Adjuvant, Freund's complete
  and cytophilic antibody production, 94-98
  and delayed sensitivity, 103, 104
  and desquamative interstitial pneumonia, 149
  and experimental allergic encephalomyelitis, 79
Alligator mississippiensis, 18
Allograft immunity, 116-121
  decrease during lepromatous leprosy, 134
  macrophages in, 118-120
  passive transfer with macrophage suspensions, 118, 119
  specific macrophage cytotoxin and, 120
  as stimulus to RES, 67
Anamnestic response
  and acquired cellular immunity, 126, 130
  and clearance of antigen, 83
Antibodies
  and acquired resistance to infection, 2, 124, 125, 128, 129, 132, 135-139, 143-146
  and allograft rejection, 120
  cytophilic (see Cytophilic antibodies)
  cytotoxic, 120
  heterogeneity of, 75, 95-99
  natural, 63, 99
  as opsonins, 60, 62-66, 69, 71-76, 93, 94, 96
  production, *in vitro,* 89-91
  production, *in vivo,* 83-89
  production, primary, 86, 87, 89-91
  production, secondary, 89-91
Antigen-antibody complexes
  and antigen clearance, 83
  cytophilia of, 98, 99
  and phagocytosis, 63
Antigens
  clearance of, by various species, 18
  competition of, 134

Antigens—*Continued*
  fate of, 83-89
  of *Mycobacterium tuberculosis,* 129
  processing by macrophages, 85-88, 104, 119, 151
  retention in lymph nodes, 99
  storage by macrophages, 88, 89
  "super-antigen," 90, 91, 129
  transfer by macrophages, 87, 88
Antilymphocyte serum, 54
Antimacrophage serum, 87
Arthus reactions, 107
Atherosclerosis, 50, 148
Autochthonous tumors, 121-123
Autoimmune diseases, 79, 123
Autophagic vacuoles, 58

BACTERIA (see Microorganisms)
Blast cells
  in allograft rejection, 117
  and cytotoxin production, 124
  and delayed sensitivity, 105, 111, 112
  and leprosy, 133, 134
  in mixed-leukocyte cultures, 39, 40, 113
  phytohemagglutinin-induced, 29, 47, 112, 133, 134
Bone marrow stem cells, 21, 22, 28

CELLULAR immunity, antimicrobial, 124-146
  cytophilic antibodies and, 100, 125, 136-139, 143-146
  delayed sensitivity and, 134, 135, 143-146
  enzyme levels of macrophages during, 45, 46, 54, 126, 127, 144
  in leprosy, 130-135
  in listeriosis, 135, 136
  lymphocytes and, 135, 136, 144-146
  passive transfer of, 135, 139
  in salmonellosis, 136, 137
  theoretical aspects of, 143-145
  in tuberculosis, 127-130

Cellular immunity, antimicrobial—*Cont.*
  ultrastructural changes in macrophages during, 139-143
Cellular immunity, anti-tissue, 115-124
  to autochthonous tumors, 121-123
  in autoimmune diseases, 123
  cytophilic antibodies and, 119-121, 123, 124
  delayed sensitivity and, 102, 103, 115
    immune macrophage-target cell interaction in, 118ff
    lymphocytes and, 117ff
    passive transfer of, 118, 119
    to Sarcoma I, 118-122
    to skin allografts, 116-119, 134
    theoretical aspects of, 123, 124
Chalones, 34
Chemotaxis, 18, 59, 111
Cholesterol, 50, 51, 55, 78, 149
Complement (C')
  and allograft immunity, 118, 120
  in antigen:antibody: C' complexes, 75, 98
  and phagocytosis, 60, 62, 63, 69, 75
  synthesis by macrophages, 19, 41, 42, 53, 120
Contact sensitivities, 102, 134
Cortisone (adrenal hormones), 42, 66, 67, 68, 128
Cytophilic antibodies, 93-100
  and acquired cellular immunity (see Cellular immunity, antimicrobial, and Cellular immunity, anti-tissue)
  and antibody production, 79
  characteristics of, 94-96
  classes of, 94-99
  cytophilic-binding reaction of, 97-99
  and delayed-type sensitivity, 95, 96, 104ff
  on dendritic cells in lymph nodes, 79
  and detoxification, 80, 81
  "early," 95, 97, 136, 137
  functions of, 99, 100
  "late," 95, 97, 136, 137
  and membrane phagocytosis, 71, 75
  as opsonins, 60, 63, 66, 71ff, 93, 94, 96
  receptors for, 30, 97-99
  significance of, 99, 100
  for spleen cells, 93
Cytotoxins
  of lymphocyte, 105, 111-114, 120, 124
  of macrophage, 120, 124

DELAYED-TYPE sensitivity
  and acquired cellular immunity, 102, 103, 115, 134, 135, 143-146
  and allograft rejection, 102, 103

Delayed-type sensitivity—*Continued*
  and cytophilic antibodies, 95, 96, 104ff
  in vitro manifestations of, 108-113
  in vivo studies, 103-108
  and inhibition of macrophage migration, 108ff
  and inhibition of macrophage spreading, 111
  and lymphocyte blast transformation, 105, 111, 112
  macrophages in, 24, 25, 101-114
  and mitosis of macrophages, 112
  passive transfer of, 105-107, 110, 115
Dendritic cells (see Macrophages, of lymph nodes)
Deoxyribonucleic acid (DNA)
  hybridization with macrophage RNA, 90
  synthesis by macrophages, 21, 22, 24, 25, 27
Dyes, vital
  Janus green, 5
  neutral red, 5, 43

ENCEPHALOMYELITIS, experimental allergic (EAE), 79, 123
Endocytosis, 59, 99
Endotoxins
  effects of RES function, 67, 68
  and fibrosis, 35
  and homeostasis of macrophages, 34, 35, 42
  and interferon production, 53
  and macrophage activation, 125
Energy sources, of macrophages, 42, 43, 58, 61, 62, 148
Enhancement (see Immunological enhancement)
Enzymes
  changes during cellular immune response, 45, 46, 54, 126, 127, 144
  chymotrypsin, 98
  ficin, 98
  of macrophages (see also Table 48, 49)
    adenosine triphosphatase, 45, 61, 62
    aminopeptidase, 46
    beta-glucuronidases, 44, 45
    cathepsin, 45
    cholesterol esterases, 44, 50, 51
    cytochrome oxidase, 46
    dehydrogenases, 44, 46
    esterases, 44, 46, 47, 53, 54, 81
    galactosidases, 48, 49, 54
    lipases, 44
    lysozyme (muramidase), 44-46, 55
    phosphatases, 44-47, 54, 142
    proteases, 44
  neuraminidase, 98

Enzymes—*Continued*
  papain, 97
  pepsin, 95
  phospholipase A, 98
  pronase, 90, 98, 129
  ribonuclease, 87, 90, 110, 129
  synthesis by macrophages, 43-49
Epithelioid cells
  and delayed sensitivity, 103, 104
  electron micrograph of, 15
  enzymes in, 49
  in granulomatous lesions, 9, 24, 126-
    128, 131, 132
  maturation of macrophages to, 14-16
  morphology, 14
  ultrastructure, 14, 15
Erythrocytes
  as antigen, 89, 90
  and antimacrophage serum, 87
  disposal of, 72-76
  phagocytosis of effete, 73
Erythropoietin, 32
Estrogens, 67

FERNANDEZ reaction, 131-135
Ferritin
  in macrophages, 72, 73
Fibroblasts
  and homeostasis, 37-39
  macrophage growth factor from, 24,
    38, 39, 42
  phagocytosis by macrophages, 53, 54
  as target cells, 120, 121
Fungi, 125, 135, 137

GIANT cells
  in antimicrobial cellular immunity,
    126, 127
  foreign-body, 14
  from human buffy-coat cultures, 29
  Langhans', 14
  maturation of macrophages to, 14, 126,
    127
  nuclei of, 14-16
  ultrastructure, 15
Glycolysis
  as energy source for peritoneal macro-
    phages, 42, 43
  during phagocytosis by macrophages,
    61
Golgi apparatus (see Macrophages, ultra-
    structure of)
Graft rejection cells, 117
Graft-versus-host reactions
  and acute allogeneic disease (AAD),
    118
  and allograft immunity, 118

Graft-versus-host reactions—*Continued*
  and RES activity, 28, 67
Granulocytes (see Polymorphonuclear
    leukocytes)
Granulomas
  and cellular immunity, 126-129
  and delayed sensitivity, 103, 104
  enzymes in macrophages of, 49, 54
  and epithelioid cells, 24, 49, 126ff
  experimental, of man, 24
  in leprosy, 131-135

HISTAMINE
  as stimulant to phagocytosis, 67
Histiocytosis, 148
Homeostasis
  general theories concerning, 31-34
  macrophages and, 34-40, 89
Hormones
  adrenal, 42, 66, 67, 68, 128
  estrogenic, 67
  monocytogenic, 35
  thyroid, 67, 127, 128
Hortega cells (see Macrophages, of cen-
    tral nervous system)
Hyaloplasmic veils
  and movement of macrophages, 5, 7

IMMUNE cell-target cell interactions
  and macrophage plaques (photograph),
    121
  of macrophages in Sarcoma I system,
    118-121, 123, 124
  theoretical aspects of, 123, 124
Immune deviation
  and delayed sensitivity, 104
  and depression of cellular immunity,
    134, 135
Immunological enhancement
  and depression of cellular immunity,
    134, 135
Immunological tolerance
  and depression of cellular immunity,
    134, 135
  and macrophage function, 87
Inflammation
  and delayed sensitivity, 101, 105
  and macrophage maturation, 24, 27-30
  and macrophage proliferation, 28
  macrophage enzymes in, 48, 49
Interferon, synthesis by macrophages, 52,
    53
Iron metabolism
  and detoxification, 81
  macrophage function and, 72-74
Irradiation
  and antigen processing by macro-
    phages, 37, 86

Irradiation—*Continued*
  chimeras, 21, 22, 28
  and delayed sensitivity, 102
  and inflammatory response, 22
  and leprosy in mice, 130
  and RES function, 37, 68, 69, 86

JERNE, plaque assay, 90

KUPFFER cells (see Macrophages, of liver)

LEPROSY, 130-135
Lipidoses, 50, 148
Lipids
  degradation by macrophages, 55
  influence on RES function, 67
  and macrophage proliferation, 34
  and metabolic diseases, 50, 148, 149
  of mycobacteria, 126
  phagocytosis of, by macrophages, 58
  phospholipid increases, 51
  removal from blood by alveolar macrophages, 78, 79
  Restim, 67
  synthesis by macrophages, 50, 51
Listeria monocytogenes
  and cellular immunity, 129, 130, 135, 136
  and monocytosis-producing agent, 34, 135
Lymph nodes
  in allograft immunity, 117
  and antibody production, 84ff
  antigen retention in, 84-89
  dendritic macrophages in, 79, 84
  and delayed sensitivity, 105, 109, 110
Lymphocytes
  and acquired cellular immunity, 117ff, 135, 136, 144-146
  and allograft immunity, 117-120
  and antimacrophage serum, 87
  blast transformation of, 29, 39, 40, 47, 105, 111, 112, 117, 124, 133, 134
  chemotactic factor produced by, 105, 106
  cytotoxin produced by, 105, 111-114, 120, 124
  and delayed sensitivity, 101, 102, 105-107, 110-114
  heterogeneity of, 28-30
  and immunity to neoplasms, 122
  migration inhibitory factor produced by, 108-114
  phagocytosis of, by macrophages, 54
  possible transformation to macrophages, 27-30, 37, 39, 40, 47
Lymphoid follicles, 84, 85

Lymphotoxin, 105, 111-114, 120, 124
Lysosomes of macrophages
  during cellular immunity, 126, 127, 140, 142
  enzymes of, 43-49, 54
  in macrophages of lymph nodes, 84
  and rheumatic diseases, 150
  ultrastructure of, 8, 9, 12, 14, 15
Lysozyme (muramidase)
  in macrophages, 44-46, 55

MACROPHAGE congregation, 78
Macrophage disappearance reaction, 106
Macrophage growth factor (MGF), 24, 38, 39, 42
Macrophage migration inhibition, 108-114
  photograph, 109
Macrophages, and acquired cellular immunity, 115-146 (see also Cellular immunity, antimicrobial, and Cellular immunity, anti-tissue)
  cytophylic antibody and, 100, 125, 128, 129, 136-139, 143-146
  enzyme levels in, 45, 46, 54, 126, 127
  in fish, 18
  during ontogeny, 19
  passive transfer, 115, 118, 119, 135-137, 144, 145
Macrophages, activation of, 7, 8, 10, 11, 14, 22, 23, 77, 79, 88, 111, 125ff
Macrophages, alveolar
  and antibody production, 94
  cigarette smoke and, 78
  compared with peritoneal, 9
  electron micrographs of, 10, 140-142
  enzymes of, 45, 46, 48, 49
  functions of, 77
  and lipid metabolism, 50, 51
  method for obtaining, 45
  morphology, 9, 10
  relation to septal cells, 25, 51
  synthesis of interferon by, 52
  ultrastructure, 9, 10
Macrophages, of bone marrow, 14, 48, 49, 73
Macrophages, of central nervous system (Microglia cells)
  and experimental allergic encephalomyelitis, 79
  function of, 79
  morphology, 13
  sources of, 26-27
  ultrastructure, 13
Macrophages, cultivation *in vitro,* 41, 42
Macrophages, definition of, 1
Macrophages, in disease
  fibrosis, 149

Macrophages, in disease—*Continued*
  infectious diseases, 147-148
  metabolic diseases, 148-149
  monocytosis, 147
  neoplasms, 150
  pathogenesis, 150-151
  silicosis, 149
Macrophages, functions of
  in acquired cellular immunity (see
    Macrophages, and acquired cellu-
    lar immunity)
  in antibody production, 83ff
  degradation of polysaccharides, 54,
    55
  in delayed sensitivity (see Delayed-
    type sensitivity)
  detoxification
    of endotoxins, 68, 81
    of exotoxins, 80
    of simple chemicals, 80, 81
  digestion of foreign materials, 2, 17,
    71ff, 84ff, 93
  disposal of effete cells, 72-74, 93
  in homeostatis, 31ff, 89
  inactivation of thromboplastin, 81
  in iron metabolism, 72-74
  as nurse cells, 79, 80
  in pathogenesis of diseases, 150, 151
  in relation to metabolic activities,
    53-55
  in RES clearance, 64ff
  resorption and reutilization of mate-
    rials, 14, 53-55, 74
  scavenger activities, 71ff
  synthesis
    of enzymes, 43ff
    of interferon, 52, 53
    of lipids, 50, 51
    of serum proteins, 53
Macrophages, immune (see also Macrophages, and acquired cellular immunity)
  desensitization of, 98, 99
Macrophages, life span of, 24-26
Macrophages, of liver (Kupffer cells)
  enzymes of, 48, 49
  functions of, 12, 61, 74-76
  in vitro characteristics of, 25, 26
  methods for obtaining, 12
  "micropinocytosis vermiformis" of,
    12, 13
  migration to lung, 25, 26
  sources of, 22, 28
  ultrastructure, 12
Macrophages, of lymph nodes
  and antibody formation, 84-86
  as dendritic cells, 79, 84

Macrophages, of lymph nodes—*Cont.*
  electron micrograph, 96
  enzymes of, 48, 49
  and lipid synthesis, 50
  as reticular cells, 79, 84
  ultrastructure, 11
Macrophages, of male reproductive organs, 14, 80
Macrophages, maturation of, 22-24 (see
  also Macrophages, activation of)
Macrophages, mitosis of
  and delayed sensitivity, 24, 25, 112,
    113
  rates of, 25, 26
  stimuli for, 24, 25, 28
Macrophages, of the ovary, 14, 48, 49,
    53
Macrophages, peritoneal
  activated, 8
  compared with alveolar, 9
  electron micrograph of, 7
  enzymes of, 44, 45, 48, 49
  functions of, 77
  immune, 8, 115ff
  and interferon synthesis 52, 53
  and lipid synthesis, 50, 51
  morphology, 7-9
  photographs of, 7, 109, 121, 122
  proliferation of, 24, 25
  and serum protein synthesis, 53
  ultrastructure, 7-9
Macrophages, in post-secretory mammary involution, 14, 74
Macrophages, of the skin, 14, 80
Macrophages, sources and proliferation
  of
  blood monocytes, 22, 23
  bone marrow stem cells, 21, 22, 28
  in delayed sensitivity, 112, 113
  division of existing macrophages, 24-
    26
  endothelium, 23
  lymphocyte transformation, 27-30
  milk spots of the omentum, 24, 27
  tissue mesenchyme, 23, 24
Macrophages, of the spleen
  energy sources of, 61
  enzymes of, 47-49
  functions of, 11, 73-76, 79, 85, 89,
    90
  ultrastructure, 11
Macrophages, substances toxic for
  endotoxins (see Endotoxins)
  silicon dioxide (silica), 36-38, 65,
    78, 119, 129, 149
  thorium dioxide (Thorotrast), 36,
    52, 65, 66, 68

Macrophages, of thymus
    function, 74
    morphology, 12
Macrophages, ultrastructure of
    during cellular immune responses,
        139-143
    endoplasmic reticulum, 6, 8, 9, 11,
        13, 14
    Golgi apparatus, 5, 8, 9, 11, 13, 15
    lysosomes 8, 9, 12, 14, 15
    mitochondria, 6-10, 12-14
    nuclei, 5-11, 13-15
    nucleoli, 6, 8, 11, 13, 14
    phagolysosomes, 8, 12, 15
    phagosomes 8-11, 15
    pinosomes, 8
    polyribosomes, 8, 14
    ribosomes, 6, 8, 11, 14
Macrophages, of the uterus, 14, 74
Macrophages, and virus infections, 52, 53,
    78, 124, 125
Malaria, 138, 139
Mast cells, in peritoneal fluids, 53
Melanophage, 14, 80
Membrane phagocytosis, 71, 73, 75, 120,
    124
    electron micrograph of, 122
Metabolic inhibitors
    and energy production, 42, 43, 61
    and interferon production, 52
    and production of migration inhibitory
        factor, 110
Metabolism of macrophages, 41-56
    energy sources, 42, 43, 58, 61, 62, 148
    enzyme synthesis, 43-49
    interferon synthesis, 52, 53
    lipid synthesis, 50, 51
    metabolic requirements in vitro, 41, 42
    protein synthesis, 19, 41, 42, 53-56
    relation to function, 53
Microglia cells (see Macrophages, of cen-
    tral nervous system)
Microorganisms
    Bacillus, 18
    Brucella, 137, 138, 147
    Corynebacterium, 28
    Coccidioides, 135
    Diplococcus, 55, 62
    Escherichia, 63, 69, 88
    Histoplasma, 135
    Leishmania, 135, 138, 139
    Listeria, 34, 129, 130, 135, 136
    Mycobacterium, 125, 127-135, 140,
        141, 142, 147
    Pasteurella, 137
    Plasmodium, 138, 139

Microorganisms—Cont.
    Salmonella, 63, 65, 84, 95, 127, 136,
        137, 147
    Shigella, 86
    Staphylococcus, 127
    as stimulus to RES, 67
    Streptococcus, 55, 85, 147
Micropinocytosis, 12, 13, 58
"Micropinocytosis vermiformis," 12, 13,
    15
Migration inhibition test, 108-114
Migration inhibitory factor (MIF), 110,
    111, 113
Milk spots of omentum, 24, 27
Mitochondria (see Macrophages, ultra-
    structure of)
Mitosis (see Macrophages, mitosis of)
Mitsuda reaction, 131-135
Monocytes, of blood
    during certain diseases, 147, 150, 151
    electron micrograph of, 6
    enzymes of, 46-49
    as immature macrophages, 22, 23, 59
    morphology, 5, 6
    movement of, 5
    stimulation of production
        by monocytogenic hormone, 35
        by monocytosis-producing agent, 34,
            135
    ultrastructure, 6
Monocytogenic hormone, 35
Monocytosis, 34, 35, 135, 147, 150, 151
Monocytosis-producing agent (MPA), 34,
    135
Multiple sclerosis, 79

NEOPLASMS
    macrophages and, 150
    macrophages in immunity to, 116, 121-
        123
    of reticuloendothelial tissue, 150
    as stimulus to RES, 67
Neutral red, 5, 43
Neutrophils (see Polymorphonuclear leu-
    kocytes (PMNs))
Nucleic acids (see Deoxyribonucleic acid
    and Ribonucleic acid)

ONTOGENY, of macrophages
    and antigen processing, 85-86
    of macrophages in human fetus, 18, 19
    of reticuloendothelial system, 18, 19
    and synthesis of complement, 19
Opsonins, 60, 62-66, 69, 71-76, 93, 94, 96
Orchitis, experimental autoimmune, 123
Osteoclasts, 19, 80
Oxidative phosphorylation, 43, 61

PERIPOLESIS, 94
Phagocytosis
  and body defense, 2
  divalent cations and, 59
  energy for, 42, 43, 61, 62
  by macrophages
    of erythrocytes, 72-76, 138
    factors that influence, 65-69
    humoral factors and, 62-66
    during infections with animal para-
      sites, 138, 139
    lipid synthesis in relation to, 60
    of lipids, 51
    and macrophage activation, 66
    and macrophage scavenger activities,
      71-76
    measurement of, 60
    mechanisms of, 58-61
    of membranes, 71, 73, 75, 120, 122,
      124
    pH and, 60
    temperature dependence of, 60
    and uptake of materials by macro-
      phages, 57, 58
Phagocytosis - promoting factors (non-
    specific)
  in eosinophils, 63
  in serum, 63
Phagolysosomes, 8, 12, 15, 140, 142
Phagosomes, 8-11, 15, 51, 139, 140
Pharmacological mediators
  and delayed sensitivity, 110, 111, 113
  and immune cell-target cell interaction,
    120
Phospholipid
  receptors for macrophage-cytophilic
    antibodies, 98
  synthesis of, 50, 51, 60
Phylogeny, of macrophages, 17, 18
Phytohemagglutinin, 29, 47, 112, 133,
    134
Pinocytosis
  of antibodies, 58
  and desensitization of macrophages, 99
  energy sources for, 42, 43
  inducers of, 57, 63
  by macrophages, 41-43, 57, 58
  micropinocytosis vermiformis, 12, 13,
    15
Pinosomes, 8
Plasma cells
  and allograft immunity, 117
  and homeostasis, 36
  and immunity to animal parasites, 138
  phagocytosis of, by macrophages, 11,
    53, 54, 74, 79
  and stem cells, 32

Polymorphonuclear leukocytes (PMNs)
  alkaline phosphatase in, 46
  chemotaxis of, 18, 59, 113
  destruction of Brucella by, 138
  genetic defects of, 130
  and glycogen transfer to macrophages,
    58, 125, 148
  metabolism of, 43, 61
  phagocytosis by, 18, 37, 51, 57, 58, 62,
    72, 74, 125
  pyrogen of, 151
  relation to inflammatory response, 24,
    76, 101, 148
  relation to lymphocyte-to-macrophage
    transformation, 28-30, 39, 40, 47,
    125
  in rheumatic diseases, 150
Pronase, 90, 98, 129
Protein synthesis, by macrophages, 19,
    41, 42, 53-56
Protozoa (see Microorganisms)
Pyrogens, endogenous, 151
Pyroninophilic cells, large (LPCs) (see
    Blast cells)

RESTIM, 67
Reticular cells
  of lymph nodes, 79, 84
  of spleen, 85
Reticuloendothelial system (RES)
  and aging, 50
  and allograft immunity, 117
  and antimicrobial cellular immunity,
    124
  blockade of, 52, 64, 65, 68, 69
  clearance by, 64, 83, 84
  and immunity to neoplasms, 123
  and lipid synthesis, 50
  measurement of function of, 63-65
  ontogeny of, 18, 19
  stimulation of
    during lepromatous leprosy, 134
    and macrophage proliferation, 28
    during rheumatic diseases, 151
Rheumatoid arthritis, 149, 150
Rhopheocytosis, 58
Ribonuclease (RNAase), 87, 90, 110, 129
Ribonucleic acid (RNA)
  and antibody production, 79, 83, 87,
    90, 91
  and blast transformation, 47
  complexed with antigen ("super-anti-
    gen"), 90, 91, 129
  and delayed sensitivity, 110
  and immunogen from Mycobacterium
    tuberculosis, 129

Ribonucleic acid (RNA)—*Cont.*
  and interferon production, 52
  messenger, 90, 91
Ribosomes, 6, 8, 11, 14
Rosettes
  and disposal of erythrocytes, 75
  electron micrograph of, 96
  as test for cytophilic antibodies, 94, 96

SARCOMA I, 118-122
Sertoli cells (see Macrophages, of male
      reproductive organs), 80
Silicon dioxide, crystalline (silica)
  and allograft rejection, 119
  and alveolar macrophages, 78
  granulomatous response to, 129
  and homeostasis, 36-38
  and RES function, 65
  in silico-proteinosis, 149
  in silicosis, 37, 38
Silver stain for macrophages, 44
Specific macrophage cytotoxin (SMC),
      120, 124
"Super-antigen," 90, 91, 129
Synovial cells, 149-150

TERMINOLOGY, used in tissue grafting,
      115
Thorium dioxide (Thorotrast), 36, 52,
      65, 66, 68

Thymectomy, and leprosy in mice, 130
Thymus-dependent lymphocytes, 107
Thyroid hormones, 67, 127, 128
Tolerance (see Immunological tolerance)
Transfer, passive
  of allograft immunity with suspensions
      of macrophages, 118, 119
  of cellular immunity with cell suspen-
      sions, 118, 119, 135, 139
  of delayed sensitivity, 105-107, 110,
      115
Transferrin
  and iron metabolism, 72
  synthesis by macrophages, 41, 53
Trypan blue, 26, 38
Trypsinization, of macrophages, 62, 75,
      97, 98, 109, 119, 120, 128, 136
Tuberculin-type skin test, 101, 102, 105,
      106, 107-109, 113, 114, 131-135
Tuberculosis (see Cellular immunity,
      antimicrobial)
Tumors (see Neoplasms)

VIRUS infections, 124, 125, 137

WOUND healing, 76

XANTHOMAS, 149

DATE DUE

FEB 25 '71			